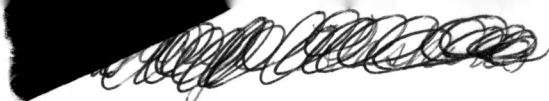

D1803747

ACUTE PSYCHIATRIC CARE

an occupational therapy
guide to exercises in
daily living skills

Patricia L. Simmons

Linda Mullins

SLACK Incorporated, 6900 Grove Road, Thorofare, New Jersey 08086

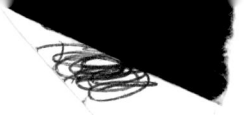

SLACK International Book Distributors

In Europe, the Middle East and Africa:
  John Wiley & Sons Limited
  Baffins Lane
  Chichester, West Sussex PO19 1UD
  England

In Canada:
  McAinsh and Company
  2760 Old Leslie Street
  Willowdale, Ontario M2K 2X5

In Australia and New Zealand:
  MacLennan & Petty Pty Limited
  P.O. Box 425
  Artarmon, N.S.W. 2064
  Australia

In Japan:
  Central Foreign Books Limited
  1-13 Jimbocho-Kanda
  Tokyo, Japan

In Asia and India:
  PG Publishing Pte Limited.
  36 West Coast Road, #02-02
  Singapore 0512

Foreign Translation Agent

  John Scott & Company
  International Publishers' Agency
  417-A Pickering Road
  Phoenixville, PA 19460

Publisher: Harry C. Benson
Managing Editor: Lynn C. Borders
Editor: Stephanie Scanlon
Designer: Susan Hermansen
Production Manager: David Murphy

Printed in the United States of America

Library of Congress Catalog Card Number: 80-54633

ISBN: 0-913590-76-2

Published by: SLACK Incorporated
              6900 Grove Rd.
              Thorofare, NJ 08086

Last digit is print number: 10 9 8 7 6 5 4

*To Paul Simmons and Gregory W. Mullins
and their families*

TABLE OF CONTENTS

ACKNOWLEDGMENTS

The authors wish to extend sincere appreciation to the following individuals for their constructive suggestions and encouragement: Elizabeth A. Boles, M.A., Associate Professor of Occupational Therapy, Wayne State University; Yvonne Teske, M.A., Assistant Professor of Occupational Therapy, Eastern Michigan University; the staff at Western Michigan University; and the staff at Henry Ford Hospital, Detroit, Michigan.

PREFACE

The needs of patients who are hospitalized in an acute psychiatric setting tend to differ in many respects from those of patients requiring long-term care. For the therapist attempting to meet these needs, time is a critical factor and priorities must be established. Identifying and dealing with problem areas must be approached realistically with emphasis on defining reasonable goals in view of the time limitation involved.

The purpose of this manual is to provide therapists working in short-term psychiatric settings with a practical tool for building essential daily living skills. While the authors have drawn on previous work experience to plan, organize, and implement the groups included in this manual, the exercises were developed and geared specifically for an adult acute psychiatric inpatient setting, representative of a broad range of diagnostic categories. Therapists are encouraged to adapt the materials to make them more suitable to individual situations, and the authors have provided some suggestions along these lines in the text.

It is the experience of the authors that this particular patient group consistently presents deficiencies in many areas of basic life skills necessary to cope effectively in the home and community environment. It has been observed that many skills improved when patients were provided the opportunity to learn about basic areas of daily living, including parenting, employment, money management, leisure planning, and assertiveness. Assisting clients in

3

preparing for discharge was also recognized as an all-encompassing major aspect of care and is included as an additional section.

While numerous references are available from libraries, community agencies, and other sources on the topics in this manual, the authors identified their own need to compile readily usable materials to facilitate group planning. As such, the authors anticipate that their fellow therapists will find this collection of exercises valuable in conducting skill-building experiences for their clients.

INTRODUCTION

A major function of occupational therapists has been the development of daily living skills, frequently referred to as life tasks. Educational curricula have long addressed some of these training needs by including courses on A.D.L. (activities of daily living), homemaking, and work simplification techniques. A dimension of life tasks that has more recently gained acceptance involves the occupational therapist functioning in the capacity of educator to foster the clients development of the survival skills necessary for independent functioning.

In both physical and psychosocial dysfunction, the trend has been toward building or improving those skills that are crucial for independent functioning in the community. While most occupational therapists have a general idea of how to apply this concept, few specific tools are available for use in the area of psychosocial dysfunction.

Gail Fidler[1] recommended a reassessment of traditional occupational therapy activities in terms of their meaningfulness in a therapeutic community, their purposefulness to the patient, and their reality in social-cultural meaning. She proposed the need for further exploration and study in the development of the role of the occupational therapist as a supportive group leader, providing the atmosphere and attitudes necessary to support the experimental daily living experiences of the patient. The uses of activities and craft media are recognized as beneficial in the psychosocial occupational therapy program; however, skill development

5

in the many areas of daily living should not be overlooked. The importance of the latter becomes most apparent when one views postdischarge adjustment: an individual may have adequately ventilated anger through the use of resistive craft media, yet he isolates himself at home because social skill development and community resources for leisure have not been explored. If occupational therapists are to meet the challenge of treating the total client, a dual approach including practical skill-building and therapeutic craft media must be attempted. No other member of the therapeutic team is as qualified as the occupational therapist to deal with the critical and fundamental issue of life task skill development.

The exercises presented in this manual attempt to develop the necessary skills through the activities therapy framework proposed by Mosey. Activities therapy is based on the assumption that psychosocial dysfunction involves poor understanding of the self and/or inability to participate in tasks of everyday life. Activities therapy correlates psychosocial dysfunction with learned maladaptive behavior; that is, the client has not learned to function adequately in the wider community. The exercises are designed to promote the development of life task skills, to prepare the individual for discharge into the community, and to prepare the individual to effectively cope with the demands of daily life.*

This manual was organized as a reference for practicing occupational therapists and as a text for occupational therapy students involved in daily living skill development. The authors have used the discussion/exercise format with a great deal of success over the past two years in an acute, psychiatric inpatient setting. The milieu unit is part of a general hospital in a large metropolitan area. This setting has therefore provided the opportunity to apply the exercises presented in this text to a wide variety of diagnostic categories. The group participants have included adult males and females covering a broad spectrum of social, cultural, and educational differences. The suitability of a

---

*Special note: Many illiterate patients have functioned well with adaptations made to include them in the groups. Often, these patients demonstrate a greater need to develop skills in many areas of daily life. Patients who cannot read or write to complete the exercises, still may be able to consider alternatives and make appropriate responses.

patient for a particular discussion group is left to the discretion of the therapist. Adaptations can be made to keep the activity within the functional level of the group. A note of caution, however — do not underestimate the patient's ability to function within the group. Individuals considered to be very withdrawn have been active participants in role playing exercises; "disoriented" participants have written realistic and meaningful plans in goal-setting exercises. Inclusion of a variety of functional levels in a group has frequently resulted in productive group discussions. The initial interview provides an excellent opportunity to define deficit areas, so that clients may be placed in the appropriate groups.

The exercises included in the manual have generally been presented in a group discussion format. In this way, the participant not only explores the specific life task skill but is given an opportunity to develop interpersonal communication skills through the group involvement. The exercises are also applicable for use as an individual treatment approach. The worksheets or cards could be completed with the client on a one to one basis or could be given as an assignment to be completed prior to discussion at the next treatment session. Another approach has been to involve a group participant in the leadership role. This has been successful with clients who have been relatively active within the groups and who would benefit from group leadership skill development.

The format of the exercises/discussions have been designed to be as straightforward as possible. Included with each exercise are goals, directions for the exercise, a suggested verbal presentation and various recommendations for adaptations. The time frame for all groups is approximately 40 minutes. Suggested group size includes eight to ten participants which should allow for sufficient variation in opinions and suggestions, maximum group productivity in terms of group participation, and yet remain within manageable limits.

Each of the exercises presented includes the use of a worksheet or situations written on 3 x 5 cards. The authors have noted that the level of group participation appears to increase when the participants are provided with a concrete exercise worksheet or card. Participants who would not generally contribute to a strictly verbal discussion appeared

to be more comfortable sharing their ideas and feelings when
the discussion was associated with a written format. In
addition to the worksheets and cards, it is recommended that
a chalkboard, clipboards for the worksheets, and pencils be
readily available to the group leader.

The worksheets are on a full page to facilitate xerox
copying of the required number of sheets for the group.
Visual limitations, often due to medications, formed the
basis for using large, dark print on the worksheets. Such
print is also recommended when copying topics and
situations onto 3 x 5 index cards.

Each exercise includes suggested adaptations. The authors
encourage the practicing therapists to modify the worksheets
or presentations in any way needed to make the discussion
more applicable to their client needs.

Although the goals and approaches to daily living skill
development groups are very different from those of
psychotherapy groups, the occupational therapist's background in individual and group dynamics will be called upon
to handle situations that arise. The therapist may be
required to use various aspects of "the self" to prepare and
effectively provide leadership for the group activities. In
Willard and Spackman's fifth edition of *Willard and
Spackman's Occupational Therapy,* the therapist's "use of
self" is defined as

> bringing together knowledge, skills, caring and basic person-
> ality strengths to help the client overcome difficulties and
> maximize abilities....the therapist may help by teaching,
> giving support, aiding in communication, engineering oppor-
> tunities for growth, confronting problems, clarifying, rein-
> forcing progress, or promoting plans for the future.

The potential areas of daily living skill development that
could be addressed are numerous. The authors have
identified the six areas of child care, use of leisure time,
employment, assertiveness, money management, and discharge preparation as the areas most frequently in need of
development in our client group. The topics are sufficiently
broad in scope so as to make them applicable over a wide
range of functional levels. The formats are simple and
concise; the approach is productive.

Therapists are encouraged to review the presentation
guidelines on page 10, as these provide an overview of the

basic format utilized throughout the manual, regardless of the topic. Within the framework of each exercise there is much room for variation. As both therapist and client increase their familiarity with the approach, the potential for these adaptations becomes more apparent. The information in the following pages has been of tremendous value to the authors in implementing an effective treatment program in an acute psychiatric setting. It is hoped that other therapists will find it a useful tool also.

References

1. Fidler GS, Fidler JW: A Communication Process in Psychiatry, Occupational Therapy. New York, The Macmillan Co, 1963, pp 140-141.
2. Mosey A: Activities Therapy. New York, Raven Press Pubs, 1973, pp 5-6.
3. Tiffany EG: Elements of the psychiatric O.T. process, in Willard and Spackman's Occupational Therapy, ed 5. Philadelphia, JB Lippincott Co, 1978, pp 296-297.

PRESENTATION GUIDELINES

1. Make the goal explicit.
2. Indicate the time involved (40 minutes). This facilitates concentration on the topic.
3. Make the group aware of the format to be used (worksheet, index cards, etc).
4. Define expectations.
5. Have something concrete for the group to relate to (worksheets, index cards, etc).
6. Maintain group control, guiding the group toward the defined goal.
7. Summarize briefly and reiterate the main points discussed.

LEISURE TIME

Introduction

The section on leisure time has been organized to focus on six subjects:

1) attitudes and motivation;

2) specific interests;

3) needs and values;

4) practical considerations, ie, money, time, physical restrictions, and energy level requirements;

5) resources;

6) social skills.

Treatment goals include the following:

1. Determination of the ways in which an individual's present method of thinking, feeling, and acting interfere with accomplishing or participating in enjoyable activities (EXERCISE I).

2. To identify specific interest areas (EXERCISE II).

3. To focus on the physiological and emotional needs relative to leisure time (EXERCISE III).

4. To look at the ways in which a person's values influence the types of activities he has chosen to participate in (EXERCISE III).

5. Exploration of a wide range of activities in terms of the energy requirement and cost involved (EXERCISES IV, V, VI).

6. To identify approximately the amount of time an individual has available for leisure (EXERCISE VII).

7. To assess and broaden an individual's awareness of his community resources (EXERCISES VIII, IX).

8. To build social skills and promote increased social interaction (EXERCISE X).

EXERCISE I

Purpose

The focus is on the concept of motivation to help individuals identify more clearly for themselves what particularly interferes with their participation in enjoyable activities. This is approached by looking at the excuses people commonly utilize to avoid activity involvement. The second step looks at the positive argument a person can use to get himself involved. Basically, every time a negative excuse is generated, it is paired with a positive argument.

Suggested
Verbal
Presentation

1. The leader begins by distributing a copy of the worksheet and introducing the topic with the following discussion: *What we would like to do is to take a look at the idea of motivation. Can anyone define this?* (Dictionary definition: motivation is a need or desire that causes a person to act.) *In an effort to see what motivates each of us for doing something, let's first look at the negative side of the picture. What are some of the excuses you use to avoid becoming involved in an activity?*

2. The leader directs the group to look at the worksheet. It should be folded along the dotted lines and placed "excuses" side up to be worked on first. Allow approximately ten minutes for this part.

3. When the group has finished with this section, the leader encourages everyone to share his ideas. These ideas are compiled on a blackboard, which serves as a visual guide for the entire group when the positive arguments are being generated.

4. The group is now directed to unfold the worksheets, and the leader continues with: *We are going to review each excuse individually and look at a positive argument that you can use to pair with each excuse. For example, a friend invites you to go to the show with him. The excuse may be, "I have*

13

too much work to do." *The positive argument might be,* "It really isn't necessary that I do it right now. It could be done later." Clarify with additional examples if necessary.

5. Each excuse is now reviewed while the group indicates the positive arguments on their worksheets next to the appropriate excuse.

6. The leader summarizes the discussion, possibly giving positive feedback for the group's participation and reiterating the main points of the topic.

Adaptations

1. Lengthen or shorten the time allotted for generating the excuses.

2. Divide the group into dyads or triads, working through the same format.

3. Each individual (or dyad) could complete both parts (excuses and positive arguments), and then share the ideas with the group.

Name _____

MOTIVATION

List Excuses You Com-
monly Use to Avoid Do-
ing an Activity:

I Can Say This to Help
Motivate Me:

1. _____

2. _____

3. _____

4. _____

5. _____

6. _____

7. _____

8. _____

9. _____

10. _____

11. _____

12. _____

13. _____

14. _____

EXERCISE II

Purpose

　　Activities of interest will be identified.

**Suggested
Verbal
Presentation**

1. The leader distributes a copy of the worksheet and begins with the following discussion: *What we would like to do is to take a look at some of the activities you have enjoyed doing in the past or that you think you might like to try in the future.*

2. The group is directed to indicate on the worksheet those activities of interest by placing a checkmark or circling the item. Draw attention to the bottom line where other activities can be written.

3. When everyone is finished, encourage the group members to share their ideas. Possible discussion questions include:

　a) How often do you participate in that?

　b) With whom do you do it?

　c) Where?

　d) How much does it cost?

4. The leader summarizes, possibly giving positive feedback for the group's participation and reiterating the main points of the topic.

Adaptations

1. Limit the number of items the group can check, ie, *Indicate your first five preferences.*

2. Read through each item, especially if the group has verbal or visual limitations.

3. Review each item individually, ie, *How many people checked swimming?* Then follow up with the discussion questions.

4. This is an excellent opportunity to draw the group's attention to community resources, and it is particularly beneficial to have specific information available (ie, recreation programs, special events, etc, for your area).

Name _____

INTEREST CHECKLIST

Check Those Activities You Have Enjoyed Doing in the Past or That You Might Like to Try in the Future:

Swimming
Table Games
Photography
Drama Groups
Discussion Groups
Choral Groups
Woodworking
Music Listening
Playing a Musical
   Instrument
Social Dancing
Pool
Sewing
Bicycling
Movies
Union Activities
Bowling
Lectures
Taking a Class
Poetry
Going to Restaurants

Political Organizations
Community Action
   Groups
Museums
Travel
Sketching/Painting
Cooking
Sculpture
Fixing Things
Watching T.V.
Casual Conversation
Gardening
Shopping
Church Groups
Sports
Volunteer Work
Other: _____

_____

_____

EXERCISE III

Purpose

This exercise focuses on the physiological and emotional needs relative to leisure time and looks at how values affect the types of activities people choose to become involved in.

Suggested
Verbal
Presentation

1. The leader distributes a copy of the worksheet and begins with the following discussion: *Let's try to identify some of the benefits of leisure. Is leisure time necessary? (If yes, why? If no, why?) What do we gain from leisure?*

2. As the group generates ideas for the discussion questions, indicate the ideas on the blackboard.

3. The group is next directed to look at the worksheet with an explanation about the four sections. Clarify if necessary and allow approximately ten minutes for completion of this section.

4. When everyone is finished, encourage the group members to share their ideas. Possible discussion questions include:

   a) What activities did you list?

   b) Why did you enjoy these?

   c) Can you repeat any of these activities? If yes, why? If no, why?

   d) If no, do you think your reasons are valid? What does the group think?

   e) Were you able to identify your values and needs about leisure? Some of the ideas we wrote on the blackboard might help you.

5. The leader summarizes, possibly giving positive feedback for group participation and reiterating the main points of the topic.

Adaptations

1. Read through each section and have the group complete it as you go.

2. Lengthen or shorten sections A and B.

3. Have the group complete only sections A and B with amplified discussion, omitting sections C and D.

Name: _____

VALUE SYSTEMS

This Exercise is Designed to Help You Identify Needs and Values About Leisure Time.

A. List the Last Three Activities You Really Enjoyed Doing:

B. Why Were These So Enjoyable?

1. _____ ⟶ { _____
{ _____

2. _____ ⟶ { _____
{ _____

3. _____ ⟶ { _____
{ _____

C. Are You Able to Repeat These Activities? ☐ Yes ☐ No
If No, Why? _____
_____

Do You Think Your Reasons For Not Being Able to Repeat the Activities Are Valid? ☐ Yes ☐ No

D. What Do You Think Your Values and Needs About Leisure Are?

1. _____   4. _____

2. _____   5. _____

3. _____

EXERCISES IV, V, VI

Purpose

The focus of this exercise is to organize a wide range of activities in terms of the energy requirement necessary to perform each one. The exercise was orginally designed to be used with worksheets IV, V, and VI together by dividing the group into three small teams, with each team completing one exercise worksheet each. (See adaptations.)

Suggested Verbal Presentation

1. The leader begins by explaining that the purpose is to take a look at the energy requirements for several activities.

2. Three leaders must be selected, and this is a good opportunity to provide recognition to specific individuals. Note also that it is an opportunity to receive attention from the group for appropriate behavior, particularly beneficial for individuals with inappropriate, attention-seeking behavior patterns.

3. Next, encourage the group to choose a leader they feel comfortable working with. The leader may have to provide some direction to certain group members.

4. Distribute a worksheet to each group leader and explain that each sheet is directed toward a different energy level.

5. Before each group begins working, it is a good idea to define each energy level in terms of a concrete example.*

6. Allow the groups approximately 15 minutes to work on their parts of the exercise.

------

*Suggested examples might include:

Activities requiring little energy expenditure: *reading.*

Activities requiring moderate energy expenditure: *walking, bowling.*

Activities requiring considerable energy expenditure: *swimming, jogging.*

21

7. When all the groups are finished, have each leader act as spokesperson for their group, sharing the ideas the group as a whole has generated.

8. Summarize, possibly by asking how people felt about working in small groups rather than individually, providing positive feedback to the leaders and group members for their participation and reiterating the main points of the topic.

Adaptation

1. Use each worksheet for a separate group discussion with the entire group. In this case, you might want to distribute individual worksheets and have each person indicate ideas before sharing them with the group.

Name: _____

ENERGY REQUIREMENTS I

Activities That Require Very Little Energy Expenditure on Your Part:	Approx. Cost
1. _____	
2. _____	
3. _____	
4. _____	
5. _____	
6. _____	
7. _____	
8. _____	
9. _____	
10. _____	
11. _____	

ENERGY REQUIREMENTS II

Name: _____

Activities That Require Moderate Energy Expenditure From You:	Approx. Cost
1. _____	
2. _____	
3. _____	
4. _____	
5. _____	
6. _____	
7. _____	
8. _____	
9. _____	
10. _____	
11. _____	

ENERGY REQUIREMENTS III

Name: _____

Activities That Require Considerable Energy Output From You:	Approx. Cost
1. _____	
2. _____	
3. _____	
4. _____	
5. _____	
6. _____	
7. _____	
8. _____	
9. _____	
10. _____	
11. _____	

EXERCISE VII

Purpose

Participants look at their typical week in an effort to identify approximately how much time is realistically available for leisure, and how this might affect the amount and kinds of activities that can be engaged in. This is a good method for determining if a person may need some structured type of involvement (ie, day care) in considering discharge plans, or if on the other extreme, they are a "workaholic" who should consider values about leisure.

**Suggested
Verbal
Presentation**

1. The leader begins by distributing the worksheet and discussing the following: *We are going to take a look at your typical week. I know that demands can vary from one week to the next, but some activities such as sleep patterns or work hours do not usually vary too much. So, as best you can, indicate* what *you might be doing and* when *if you were home this week.*

2. It is often helpful for the leader to demonstrate on the blackboard what his schedule tends to look like, or to use a hypothetical example. Allow approximately 15 minutes for the group to complete their schedules.

3. When everyone has finished, the leader asks the following discussion questions:

   a) Who found that they have little or no time for leisure activities?

   b) Who found they have too much time for leisure, to the extent that they have very little to do and tend to be bored?

   c) Did anyone find that their schedule leaves adequate room for a sufficient but not excessive amount of leisure time?

d) Those of you who have little or no time for leisure, is there any realistic way you can adjust your schedule? If no, why? If yes, how? Does the group have any suggestions?

e) Those of you who have too much time on your hands, how can you deal with this? Does the group have any ideas?

f) Those of you who have an adequate amount of time for leisure, how do you spend your time?

4. The leader summarizes, providing positive feedback to the group for participation and reiterating the main points of the topic.

Adaptations

1. Work individually with this exercise, particularly with lower functioning clients.

2. This is a good opportunity to educate the group about community resources by having specific information available. This can be incorporated into the discussion part.

SCHEDULING TIME

Name: _____

A Typical Week's Schedule

	SUN.	MON.	TUES.	WED.	THUR.	FRI.	SAT.
6:00							
7:00							
8:00							
9:00							
10:00							
11:00							
12:00							
1:00							
2:00							
3:00							
4:00							
5:00							
6:00							
7:00							
8:00							
9:00							
10:00							
11:00							
12:00							
1:00							
2:00							
3:00							
4:00							
5:00							

EXERCISE VIII

Purpose

An individual's awareness of the resources† in his immediate community area, defined as the immediate neighborhood, is assessed. The emphasis is on whether a person's activity is truly limited by the environment or by poor use of available resources.

Suggested Verbal Presentation

1. The leader distributes the worksheet and begins with the following discussion: *What we would like to do is to take a look at your immediate neighborhood and the types of resources you have available to you. We will do this by having each of you draw a map.*

2. The leader explains the format of the worksheet, and then directs the group to indicate several north-south streets (demonstrate on the blackboard), followed by the east-west streets (demonstrate on blackboard).

3. When everyone has completed this part, take some time to list various resources on the blackboard.

4. Now direct the group to indicate various resources on their maps at the appropriate locations. It is a good idea to demonstrate a hypothetical example on the blackboard.

5. When everyone is finished, the leader asks the following discussion questions:

   a) Who found that their neighborhood has very few resources? How do you handle this?

   b) Who found that their neighborhood actually has many resources available to them? How often do you take advantage of these?

---

†*Resources, as used here, refer to the broader range of available community services, facilities, or agencies. Examples include shopping centers, banks, parks, hospitals, etc. "Activity" refers to any effort in which an individual may engage. See Adaptations for additional ideas.*

29

c) Who found that their neighborhood has some but not many resources available to them?

6. The leader summarizes, possibly by commenting about how the environment affects the types and amounts of activities people take part in and by providing positive feedback to the group for participating.

Adaptations

1. Limit or expand the definition of "immediate neighborhood" (ie, three streets over, eight streets over).

2. If time is a problem, divide the exercise into two sections:

Section One: List resources and do map. Assign the task of filling in the resources on the map outside of group time.

Section Two: Emphasis is on discussion of the maps with greater focus on the types and amounts of activity engaged in.

3. Limit resources to only those of a recreational nature or include the broad spectrum of resources. It is possible to incorporate discussion questions about daily living skills.

IMMEDIATE NEIGHBORHOOD RESOURCES

Name: _____

Your Immediate Neighborhood

```
                    |
                    |
                    |
                    |
                    |
                    |
                    |
                    |
 _____| _____ _____
|  Home  |
 _____| _____ _____
                    |
                    |
                    |
                    |
                    |
                    |
                    |
```

EXERCISE IX

Purpose

This exercise is similar to that of Exercise VIII, but Exercise IX assesses an individual's awareness of the larger community area (ie, the Detroit area) to help him become more aware of available resources.

**Suggested
Verbal
Presentation**

1. The leader distributes the worksheet and begins with the following discussion: *What we would like to do is to take a look at your community and the kinds of resources available to you. Generally, we can define your community as the area in which you live, work, and pursue entertainment. This is a broader area, as opposed to your smaller neighborhood.* Clarify this more if necessary with examples.

2. Direct the group's attention to the worksheet and explain that they are to indicate only entertainment (recreational) resources. Again, these should be in the approximate location relative to their homes. It may be necessary to clarify with a specific hypothetical example on the board. Allow approximately ten minutes for completion of this part.

3. When everyone is finished, have the group members share their maps with the group. Encourage discussion about the resources. Identify those group members who live in relatively the same areas, comparing resources, adding additional ones that might have been omitted. It is important that the leader be well acquainted with available resources.

4. The leader summarizes, possibly providing positive feedback about group participation and reiterating the main points of the topic.

Adaptations

1. Have the group list the broader spectrum of resources

rather than limiting it to those of a recreational nature. In this case, you can generate questions about daily living skills.

2. Initially identify where each person lives and have the group work in dyads or triads to put together a map.

COMMUNITY RESOURCES

Name: _____

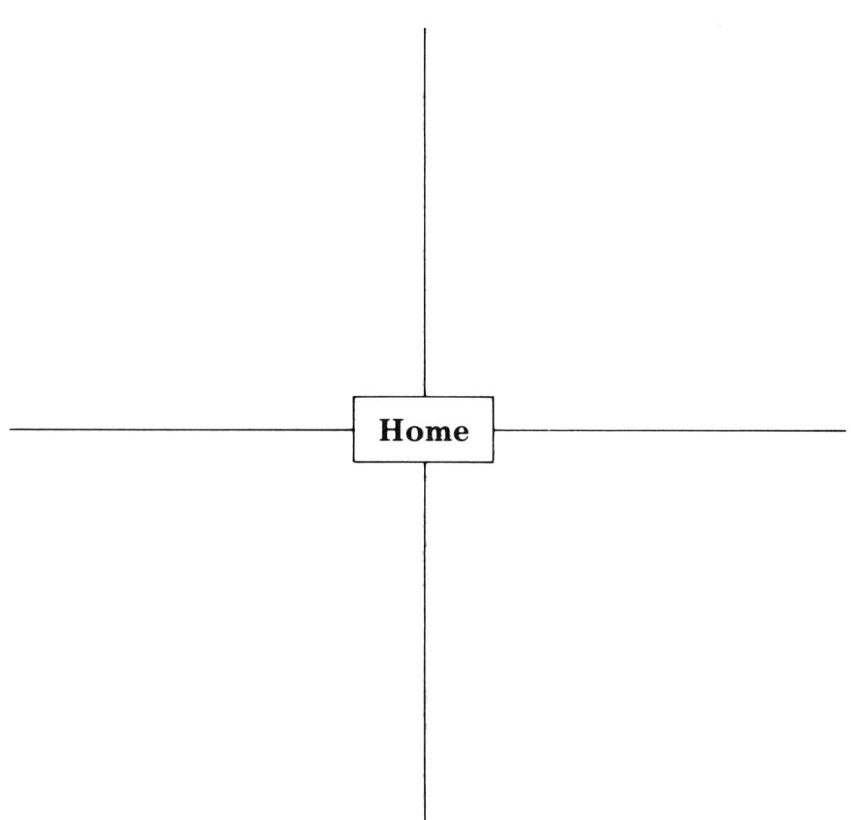

EXERCISE X

Purpose

Social skills are built by exploring what are generally considered to be appropriate items of conversation in interacting with a new acquaintance.

Suggested
Verbal
Presentation

1. The leader begins by distributing a worksheet and directing the group to indicate what they consider to be appropriate items of conversation to discuss with a person they have just met. The group is to ignore the columns to the right of the page at this time. Allow approximately ten minutes for completion of this part.

2. When everyone has finished, encourage the group members to share their ideas. The ideas can be written on the blackboard, with the leader checking for group consensus about each idea.

3. The leader directs the group members' attention to the columns at the right of the page and instructs them to check the appropriate column after each item they have written.

4. After every item has been reviewed, the leader divides the group into dyads and instructs each member to get to know their partner, following the items discussed as being appropriate in this situation. Allow approximately ten minutes for this part.

5. At the end of this time, each person is asked to talk about some of the things he has learned about his partner. Discussion can focus on people's feelings about participating in the exercise.

6. The leader summarizes, possibly by providing positive feedback to the group for participating and reiterating the main point of the topic, including the importance of taking the initiative in meeting new people.

Adaptations

1. The exercise can be done in two sections:

   Section One: Focus on appropriate conversation items.

   Section Two: Do the practice dyad, then change partners and do another sequence.

2. Assignment: Have each person take the initiative to make a new acquaintance on a daily basis (or whatever designated period of time) and discuss the outcome at the next group.

BUILDING SOCIAL SKILLS

Name: _____

List What You Think Are Appropriate Conversation Items With a Person You Have Just Met:

	Did the Group Agree with You?	
	Yes	No
1. _____		
2. _____		
3. _____		
4. _____		
5. _____		
6. _____		
7. _____		
8. _____		
9. _____		
10. _____		
11. _____		

PARENTING

Introduction

The exercises in this section address the complex role of parenting. The exercises focus upon problem identification, approaches to discipline, parent-child communication, and the use of good judgment when planning activities or purchasing toys for children.

Treatment goals include the following:

1. To identify specific problems related to child care (EXERCISE I).

2. To assess a parent's current approaches to discipline (EXERCISE I).

3. To present and explore alternative approaches to discipline (EXERCISES I, VI).

4. To promote effective communication between the parent and child (EXERCISES V, X).

5. To develop the ability to structure or plan appropriate activities for parent and/or child in a variety of situations (EXERCISES II, III, IV, IX).

6. To increase awareness of resources available in the community which are related to parenting (EXERCISES II, III, VI, VII).

7. To improve the ability to evaluate and select toys, games, and activities for children (EXERCISES VII, VIII).

EXERCISE I

Purpose

The focus is on the identification of specific parenting issues related to child care to determine what resources and methods the parent is currently using to approach problem areas. This exercise includes the completion of a problem checklist.

Suggested Verbal Presentation

1. The group leader distributes the checklist to the group participants and introduces the topic with the following discussion: *In order to determine which topics are most appropriate to focus upon in the parenting discussions, it is important to identify the aspects of child care that are problems for you. This checklist includes a number of problem areas that are common to parents. Put a check (√) in front of each problem that you have been recently confronted with.* The participants may also be instructed to list other problem areas related to parenting on the back of the worksheet.

2. When the participants have completed the exercise, the leader encourages group members to discuss the problem areas that they have identified. Possible discussion questions include:

   a) Which problem areas have you been confronted with?

   b) Which areas have been a problem in your family?

The group leader proceeds until all participants have shared their checklist results.

3. In order to assess the parent's present approach to a problem, the following discussion questions may be included:

   a) How have you been dealing with this problem?

   b) How long has this been a problem area?

c) Which approaches to this problem have been most successful for your family?

d) Which approaches have been unsuccessful?

e) Has anyone else in the group managed this problem in a different manner? If yes, what were the results?

f) Have you completely resolved any of the problems?

4. Specific suggestions for alternative approaches may be sought from other group members (as in discussion question five) or suggestions may be provided by the group leader.

5. The leader summarizes, possibly providing positive feedback for group participation, and reiterates the main points of the discussion.

Adaptations

1. The participants could be instructed to indicate the name(s) and age(s) of each child associated with the problem area.

2. When discussion of the checklist is initiated, the group leader could approach each problem area individually, asking those who have identified the item as a problem to discuss their approaches.

PROBLEM IDENTIFICATION

Name: _____

Place a Check (√) by any Problem Area that Applies to Your Situation with Your Children — Write any Additional Problems on the Back of the Sheet:

1. _____ Stealing
2. _____ Poor Parent/Child Communication
3. _____ Curfew Violation
4. _____ Poor Eating Habits
5. _____ Drugs/Alcohol
6. _____ Smoking Cigarettes
7. _____ Demanding Attention
8. _____ Temper Tantrums
9. _____ Isolation
10. _____ Demanding Things (Clothes, Toys, etc)
11. _____ Problems with School
12. _____ Arguing/Fighting with Siblings
13. _____ Refusal to Help with Household Chores
14. _____ Refusal to Return Home from School on Time
15. _____ Boredom
16. _____ Sexual Acting Out
17. _____ Refusal to Keep Room Clean
18. _____ Talking Back
19. _____ Lack of Trust
20. _____ Too Much Independence

EXERCISE II

Purpose

The parent is assisted in planning activities and structuring time to be spent with his/her children in a variety of settings, in considering the time and supplies required for the planned activity, and in increasing awareness of activities suitable for parents and children. This exercise includes the completion of a worksheet.

Suggested Verbal Presentation

1. The group leader distributes the worksheet and explains the directions with the following discussion: *This worksheet is to help you to plan specific activities for you and your children. In the first column, list three activities that you might do with your children. In the first box, indicate one indoor (home) activity. In the second box, indicate an outdoor (home) activity. In the third box, indicate an activity you could do away from home.* Allow five to ten minutes for the completion of the first column.

2. After the participants have completed column one, the leader instructs the group to write the time requirements for each activity in the boxes in column two. Allow two to five minutes for the completion of the second column.

3. After the participants have completed the second column, the leader directs the group to list any supplies required (or cost involved) for the activities in the third column. Allow two to five minutes for completion.

4. When all group participants have completed the exercise the leader encourages discussion of activities and their time and supply requirements. The following questions may be included:

   a) What indoor activity would you like to do with your children at home?

   b) What was your idea for an outdoor activity at home?

c) What would you like to do with your children away from your home?

d) How much time does this activity require? Is your time spent actively involved with your children, supervising the activity or observing the activity?

e) What supplies are needed to participate in the activity or how much would it cost to do it?

f) What ages are the children you would plan this for?

g) Would this activity be most interesting for you, your child/children, or both?

5. The group leader summarizes, possibly providing positive feedback for group participation, and reiterates the main points of the discussion.

Adaptations

1. A resource list consisting of magazine articles, books, local activity programs, local museums, libraries, park facilities, etc, could be provided after the discussion.

2. Directions for the entire worksheet could be given at one time.

3. The worksheet could be given to a small task group rather than to individuals. In this case, the group may complete the entire worksheet or may be given the task of focusing on one area.

PLANNING ACTIVITIES WITH YOUR CHILDREN

	Activity	Time	Supplies
Indoor Home			
Outdoor Home			
Away from Home			

EXERCISE III

Purpose

Participants focus on structuring activities to do with children on a seasonal basis. (Use of this exercise is appropriate for some geographic areas). This exercise includes the completion of a worksheet.

Suggested Verbal Presentation

1. The group leader explains the purpose of the activity after distributing the worksheet. The following discussion may be used: *Spending time with your children is a very important part of parenting. After completing this exercise, we will share ideas for activities you have done or would like to do with your children. The worksheet includes both indoor and outdoor activities for each season. Although the weather does not affect the indoor activities as much as those performed outdoors, the seasons may inspire indoor activities related to holidays, school activities, vacations, etc.* The leader directs the participants to look at the worksheet and instructs them to list three to five indoor and three to five outdoor activities for each season. Allow 10 to 15 minutes for the completion of the worksheet.

2. When all participants have completed the worksheet, the group leader encourages discussion and sharing of ideas. The following discussion questions may be included:

   a) What indoor activities would you like to do with your children during the (season) ?

   b) What outdoor activities would you like to do with your children during the (season) ?

   c) What age group is this activity appropriate for?

   d) What are the necessary supplies?

   e) Have you ever done this activity with your children?

3. After all participants have shared their plans or suggestions, the leader may provide a resource list of local facilities appropriate for family involvement.

4. The group leader summarizes, possibly provides positive feedback for group participation, and reiterates the focal points of the discussion.

Adaptations

1. This exercise may be done in small task groups with each group focusing on a specific season. Ten to twelve suggestions may be required for each season.

SEASONAL ACTIVITIES

Indoor Fall

Outdoor Fall

Indoor Winter

Outdoor Winter

Indoor Spring

Outdoor Spring

Indoor Summer

Outdoor Summer

EXERCISE IV

Purpose

Participants focus on structuring activities for a child which do not involve the parent or direct supervision of the parent. This exercise includes the completion of a worksheet.

Suggested
Verbal
Presentation

1. The group leader distributes the worksheet to the group, explains the purpose of the activity, and provides directions for the completion of the worksheet. The following discussion may be used: *There are times when parents would like to spend time with a child, but have other household duties which must be completed. This worksheet is a schedule which you are to complete by indicating what activities you would plan for the child for each block of time. Remember that you will be at home also but will not be able to directly participate in the activities with the child. Try to plan the child's day so that he/she will not become bored or interfere with your household tasks.* Allow 10 to 20 minutes for the completion of the worksheet.

2. When all participants have completed the exercise, the leader encourages discussion of daily plans. The following discussion questions may be included:

a) What age group did you plan the schedule for?

b) What will your child's day include?

c) Will your child require rest periods?

d) Are there household activities that the child could assist you with?

e) Where will your child be when engaged in this schedule?

f) Is your child capable of scheduling his/her own day off?

g) Would you involve your child in making plans for the day?

3. After each participant shares their plan, the leader summarizes, provides feedback for group participation, and reiterates the main points of the exercise.

Adaptations

1. In order to focus on the parent's ability to structure his/her own time as well as time for a child, the exercise could be divided into two columns, one indicating what the parent would be doing and one indicating what the child would be doing.

2. Small task groups could be formed, each planning a schedule for a specific age group.

STRUCTURING YOUR CHILD'S DAY

You will be at home, but busy all day. Your child has a day off from school. Plan the day's activities for him/her.

Time:	Activity:
8:30 - 9:00 AM	
9:00 - 9:30 AM	
9:30 - 10:00 AM	
10:00 - 10:30 AM	
10:30 - 11:00 AM	
11:00 - 11:30 AM	
11:30 - 12:00 PM	
12:00 - 12:30 PM	
12:30 - 1:00 PM	
1:00 - 1:30 PM	
1:30 - 2:00 PM	
2:00 - 2:30 PM	
2:30 - 3:00 PM	
3:00 - 3:30 PM	
3:30 - 4:00 PM	
4:00 - 4:30 PM	
4:30 - 5:00 PM	
5:00 - 5:30 PM	
5:30 - 6:00 PM	

EXERCISE V

Purpose

Children's feelings are identified in a given situation by listening to and evaluating the child's verbalizations. The long-term goal of this exercise is to improve parent-child communication skills.

Suggested
Verbal
Presentation

1. The group leader distributes the worksheet and introduces the topic with the following discussion: *Children and parents communicate through the use of words and gestures. Very often, a child cannot put his feelings into words; therefore, a parent must learn to listen carefully to understand what feelings a child is attempting to express.* The group leader explains that the exercise is to practice listening to a child's feelings. The group is instructed to read each of the ten statements made by a child and to write the feeling they think the child is trying to express. The feeling should be written in one or two words. (Some possible responses are indicated on a separate sheet.) Allow 10 to 15 minutes for the completion of the worksheet.

2. When the group members have completed the exercise, the leader encourages discussion of the feelings perceived in each individual situation. The following discussion questions may be included:

a) What do you think the child was feeling in this situation?

b) How might you respond to the child's feelings?

c) Have any of your children expressed similar feelings? If yes, how did you respond? Do you think you responded to the child's words or to the child's feelings?

d) Who would respond to this situation in a different manner than those already suggested?

e) What examples could you give that relate to a time when your child expressed specific feelings? (It was through this question that the suggested situations were derived. Other examples may be found in the references.)

3. The group leader may verify answers or supply suggestions as necessary.

4. After all group participants have shared their ideas and answers, the group leader summarizes, possibly providing positive feedback for group participation, and reiterates the importance of recognizing feelings in the communication process.

Adaptations

1. The verbalizations of the child could be tape recorded or written on 3 x 5 cards to encourage more group interaction.

2. Prior to beginning the worksheet, the group could be instructed to brainstorm all the possible feelings that a child might express.

3. This exercise could be written to focus upon feelings expressed by adults to encourage improvement in a broader range of communication skills.

PARENT-CHILD COMMUNICATION

Name: _____

1. Look mommy. I'm giving my new doll a bath.

    1. _____

2. I wish I had something to do. I'm tired of watching TV.

    2. _____

3. All the other kids went to school. I wish I was old enough.

    3. _____

4. Tommy is so mean. I'm never going to play with him again.

    4. _____

5. I'm glad you're my daddy.

    5. _____

6. I wish I hadn't pushed Lisa down. Am I bad?

    6. _____

7. Will you stay with me when I go to the dentist?

    7. _____

8. I'd like to ask Susan to go to the dance but what if she says no or laughs at me?

    8. _____

9. What's the use? Everytime I do my homework I get a C.

    9. _____

10. Wow! Only three more days until we go on vacation!

    10. _____

Suggested answers for feelings worksheet.

1.	Proud	Pleased
2.	Bored	Stumped
3.	Lonely (left behind)	Jealous
4.	Angry	Hurt
5.	Proud	Grateful
6.	Guilty	Sorry
7.	Afraid	Insecure
8.	Afraid	Anxious
9.	Frustrated	Inadequate
10.	Excited	Anxious

EXERCISE VI

Purpose

To introduce the concept of making changes in a child's surroundings as an approach to changing unacceptable behavior, to identify specific changes which could be made, and to provide resources for further exploration of changes.

Suggested Verbal Presentation

1. The group leader distributes the worksheet and introduces the exercise with the following discussion: *When a child is very young, we frequently make changes in the home to prevent accidents or mischief. Such changes could also prevent unacceptable behavior throughout childhood and adolescence. By preventing unacceptable behavior before it occurs, the necessity to reprimand decreases.* The leader directs the participants to look at the worksheet. *The sheet is divided into eight categories of changes that could be made.§ For each of the categories, list three things that you could change in your home that might eliminate an unacceptable behavior in one or more of your children.* The leader instructs the group that each category will be discussed. Beginning with section one, the leader briefly defines the approach and allows two to three minutes for completion of that section.

2. When participants have completed section one, the leader encourages sharing ideas. The following discussion questions may be used:

a) What changes could you make in your home to enrich the environment?

b) How would you expect your child to respond to this change?

c) Have you tried to make such changes before? What were the results?

_____

§*Gordon T: P.E.T., Parent Effectiveness Training. New York, New American Library, 1975.*

3. The leader continues to introduce each category, allows time for completion of the section, and encourages discussion of each approach.

4. After each of the eight approaches are discussed, the group leader summarizes, possibly offering positive feedback for group participation, and reiterates the main points of the exercise.

Adaptations

1. In addition to the examples provided on the worksheet, additional suggestions could be given at the end of the discussion of each category. Additional suggestions could be outlined on a supplementary handout.

2. Directions for the entire worksheet could be given, allowing 10 to 15 minutes for the task completion with discussion to follow.

3. Small task groups could be assigned to consider one or two of the categories, writing as many possible changes as the group can think of.

4. An additional assignment could be given to list specific problem areas and to list changes which could be made to alleviate the problem. A worksheet is included for this approach.

CHANGING BEHAVIOR BY
CHANGING THE ENVIRONMENT

Name: _____

I. *Enriching* — providing child with interesting and
challenging activities.
1. Supplies for quiet activities
(playing cards, fingerpaints)

     a. _____

     b. _____

     c. _____

2. Supplies/areas for physical activities
(swing, tricycle)

     a. _____

     b. _____

     c. _____

3. Time for activities away from home
(picnic, museum)

     a. _____

     b. _____

     c. _____

II. *Impoverishing* — reducing stimulation (particularly at bedtime, mealtimes)
(limiting the amount of TV)

     a. _____

     b. _____

     c. _____

III. *Simplifying* — making it easier for the child to do things for himself
   (putting closet hooks at a low level)

      a. _____

      b. _____

      c. _____

IV. *Restricting* — limiting life space
   (fenced in yard)

      a. _____

      b. _____

      c. _____

V. *Childproofing* — removing unsafe items or things which you don't want the child to have
   (locking up medicines)

      a. _____

      b. _____

      c. _____

VI. *Substituting* — offering the child an alternative before taking something away
   (substituting an old magazine for your new book)

      a. _____

      b. _____

      c. _____

VII. *Planning Ahead* — letting the child know in advance what will be happening to him
    (talking about a scheduled dentist appointment)

        a. _____

        b. _____

        c. _____

VIII. *Making Arrangements With Older Children* —
    (providing alarm clocks, discussing curfews)

        a. _____

        b. _____

        c. _____

ASSIGNMENT SHEET

List conflict areas that you are having (Column 1). List any environmental changes that you could make to resolve the problem.

Problem Area	Change

EXERCISE VII

Purpose

Participants focus upon the importance of good judgment when purchasing a child's toy. Small task groups have the opportunity to evaluate toys through the use of a worksheet. One toy per task group should be available for evaluation.

Suggested
Verbal
Presentation

1. The leader divides the group into small task groups with two to three persons per group. The leader distributes one worksheet per group and instructs each task group to appoint a recorder to fill out the worksheet. The leader introduces the task with the following discussion: *Purchasing a toy is a routine practice with many parents. Frequently, toys are purchased because the child wants it and no careful consideration is given to the safety and practicality of the toy. This exercise is to practice looking at a toy objectively in terms of its safety, learning value, durability, cost, and age appropriateness. It is hoped that after completion of this exercise you will have a better idea of what to look for when purchasing toys for your children.*

2. The leader provides each group with a different toy and instructs the group to complete the questionnaire. The leader informs the groups that they will discuss their results with the total group upon completion. Allow 12 to 15 minutes for the completion of the exercise.

3. After all groups have completed the evaluation worksheet, each group is encouraged to present their toy and the evaluation worksheet results. Discussion questions may include:

   a) Are there any other safety considerations which this group did not report?

   b) What other reasons are there for buying this toy?

   c) What could a child learn from this toy?

d) Would you purchase this toy for your children?

e) Do you ordinarily consider these factors when purchasing a toy for your child?

f) What other factors do you consider?

4. After all groups have presented their evaluations and have shared the results, the group summarizes, possibly providing positive feedback for group participation, and reiterates the importance of good judgment when selecting a child's toy.

Adaptations

1. In a small group, each participant could be given a toy to evaluate.

2. The leader could present one toy and each participant could evaluate the same toy on an individual basis.

3. An example could be provided by the group leader.

4. Local toy stores or toy departments of large department stores frequently distribute pamphlets outlining safety features and other aspects of toy selection. Such resources could be made available to the group.

GAME/TOY EVALUATION WORKSHEET

Name: _____

1. Age Group the Toy is Appropriate for: _____

2. Safety Considerations: _____
   _____
   _____
   _____

3. Why Would This Toy Be Good for a Child?
   _____
   _____
   _____
   _____

4. Is This an Indoor or an Outdoor Toy? _____

5. Does Playing with This Toy Require Adult Supervision? _____

6. Does the Toy Make Excessive Noise? _____

7. How Long Will the Toy Last? _____

8. Approximately How Much Does the Toy Cost? _____

EXERCISE VIII

Purpose

Awareness of age appropriate toys and games for children is increased. This exercise includes the completion of a worksheet.

Suggested
Verbal
Presentation

1. The group leader distributes the worksheets to each participant and introduces the topic with the following discussion: *Very often, toys are purchased for children because they express an interest in them after seeing advertisements on television or in magazines. Frequently, little thought is given to the suitability of a toy or game to the child's age. This exercise is to help identify what types of toys and games are appropriate for particular age groups.*

2. The participants are instructed to complete the worksheet, identifying three toys or games for each age group. Allow 10 to 15 minutes for completion of the task.

3. When the participants have completed the worksheet, discussion may be facilitated by the following questions:

a) What types of toys or games do you feel are appropriate for (age group) ?

b) Do you have any children in this age group? If yes, what kinds of games and toys do they seem to like?

c) If your child wanted a particular toy, how would you determine if it was appropriate for his/her age?

4. After each age group is discussed, the group leader reiterates the main points of the discussion and provides positive feedback for group participation.

Adaptations

1. Information published by toy companies or toy stores

could be distributed to the group to assist with determination of age suitability of the toys.

2. A list of 15 toys or games could also be compiled and a written exercise be used to match the toy with the appropriate age.

3. A developmental scale such as the one in the AOTF Publication "Watch Me Grow" serves as an excellent resource for the parent to refer to when completing this exercise.

AGE APPROPRIATE TOYS AND GAMES

Name: _____

1. List three toys which are suitable for an infant.

    a. _____

    b. _____

    c. _____

2. List three toys which are suitable for a pre-schooler.

    a. _____

    b. _____

    c. _____

3. List three toys which are suitable for a 6 to 8-year-old.

    a. _____

    b. _____

    c. _____

4. List three toys which are suitable for a 10-year-old.

    a. _____

    b. _____

    c. _____

5. List three toys/games which are suitable for a pre-teenager.

    a. _____

    b. _____

    c. _____

EXERCISE IX

Purpose

Participants focus upon increasing the ability to make spontaneous decisions required in planning activities for a child in a variety of situations. This exercise includes the use of situations written on 3 x 5 index cards.

Suggested
Verbal
Presentation

1. The group leader displays the situation cards and explains that they will be used to discuss making plans for a child or children. The following discussion may be used: *Day to day situations arise which require decisions and planning related to child care. These cards include situations which require action on your part to plan or suggest ideas for activities for the child or children in the situation. Each person will select a card, read it aloud to the group, and respond to the situation. Others may add their suggestions afterward.*

2. The leader distributes each card individually and encourages responses and discussion. The following discussion questions may be used:

a) What would you do if you were in this situation?

b) Have you ever been in a similar situation with your child? What did you do?

c) Are there any other suggestions of handling this situation?

3. After all situations are discussed, the leader reiterates the main points and provides feedback for group participation.

Adaptations

1. Additional situations could be added which may have been identified as problem areas by the parent or which may have been only briefly discussed in other exercises.

ACTIVITY PLANNING SITUATIONS

The following situations should be written on individual 3 x 5 cards to be used in the discussion.

1. Your 9-year-old is complaining that he cannot do his math homework and wants to watch television instead.

2. Your 7-year-old only had a half day of school today. You would like to spend more time with the child but he/she wants to play with friends.

3. It is a Saturday afternoon and it has been raining all day. Your children, ages 7, 9, and 11 watched television all morning and are asking you what they can do now.

4. You are planning a birthday party for your 7-year-old. What could you do to keep them entertained?

5. Your 12-year-old son has been ill for the past few days. The doctor says he should stay at home for five more days but does not need to stay in bed. What could you suggest for him to do?

6. Your children have two weeks vacation over a holiday. Usually, they are complaining about being bored by the second day. What plans could you make with them?

EXERCISE X

Purpose

Communication skills between parent and child are improved through the use of role play. Suggestions for situations may be contributed from the group or may be selected from those included in this exercise.

Suggested Verbal Presentation

1. The group leader displays the situation cards and explains the purpose of the group. The following discussion may be used: *In order to improve your ability to communicate effectively with your children we are going to practice our responses to the situations written on each card. Each person will select a card and then select a partner to be the other person in the situation.* After a pair has had a chance to role play the situation, others may share ways to handle the situation differently.

2. The group leader encourages someone to select the first card and clarifies the situation if necessary. After each situation, the leader promotes discussion of alternatives. The following discussion questions may be used:

   a) Would anyone respond to this situation differently?

   b) Has anyone been faced with a similar situation? How did you manage the situation?

   c) Do you feel that the presented responses would be effective in communicating with your child?

3. After discussion of all situations, the group leader summarizes the importance of parent-child communication, provides positive feedback for group participation, and encourages the members to practice the communication skills when dealing with their children.

Adaptations

1. Situations could be written based on problems identified in Exercise I.

70

ROLE-PLAY SITUATIONS

The following situations should be written on 3 x 5 index cards if used as a basis for role play and discussion in this exercise.

1. It is necessary for your 5-year-old to be admitted to the hospital for three to four days to have his tonsils removed. Prepare him for the hospital visit.

2. Your 12-year-old brought home his/her first honor roll report card.

3. You have discovered your 6-year-old playing with matches in the laundry room.

4. Your 7-year-old has been refusing to eat dinner for the past week.

5. Your mother seems to be spoiling your child with excessive gifts.

6. Your 4-year-old cut his/her hand on an old can he/she found in the yard.

7. Your 10-year-old daughter has asked if she can join the girl scouts.

8. The school principal has asked you to talk to your 16-year-old about his poor grades.

9. Your 2-year-old is having a temper tantrum in the grocery store because he/she wants some candy.

10. Your child is asking questions about why you and your spouse are getting a divorce.

Bibliography‡

Comer JP, Pouissant F: Black Child Care. New York, Pocket Books, (Division of) Simon & Schuster, 1976.

Dinkmeyer D, McKay GD: Systematic Training for Effective Parenting. Circle Pines, Minn, American Guidance Service Inc, 1976.

Ginott HG: Between Parent and Child. New York, Macmillan Co, 1976.

Gordon T: P.E.T. In Action. New York, Bantam Books, 1976.

Gordon T: P.E.T., Parent Effectiveness Training. New York, New American Library, 1975.

Granger RH: Your Child From One To Six. U.S. Department of Health, Education, and Welfare, Publication No (OHDS) 78-300026.

Hallem JF, Vermier J: 50 things for kids to do when they say "Mommy, I'm bored." Family Circle 91:106, 1978.

Harrison-Ross P, Wyden B: The Black Child. New York, Peter H. Wyden Inc, 1973.

---

‡*Other Resources Which May Be Available To The Group Leader Include:*

City Recreation Department Directory

Local Community Center Activity Programs

Local Field Trip Directory

Local Cooperative Extension Services

Parent Clubs

Youth Assistance Programs

Adult Education Programs (contact Child Development Coordinator)

Parents Magazine

Parent Effectiveness Training Instructors

Various brochures are available from several vendors of child-related products

ASSERTIVENESS TECHNIQUES

Introduction

The exercises in this section of the manual address the issue of assertiveness. It is recommended that the therapist be familiar with the material listed in the references and able to summarize background information and basic principles of assertion. Participation in an organized Assertiveness Training Program by qualified personnel is recommended.

Practice of assertiveness techniques in the structured situations provided by these exercises may help the participant to overcome anxiety about being assertive and begin to develop the social skill of self-expression, possibly improving self-esteem. The writers do not see these exercises as an assertiveness training program but as a tool to increase awareness of assertion, to increase awareness of feelings and responses to situations requiring assertiveness, and to begin to develop a repertoire of assertive behavior.

Treatment goals include the following:

1. To define assertive responses through definition and examples, contrasting assertion with aggression and nonassertion (EXERCISE I).

2. To increase awareness of behavior and level of comfort in situations which call for assertiveness (EXERCISES II, IV).

3. To develop the ability to state needs and feelings in a direct, assertive manner (EXERCISES III, IV).

EXERCISE I

Purpose

Background information on the topic of assertiveness is provided by defining assertive behavior, contrasting assertion with nonassertion and aggression, and by providing examples of the different responses. This exercise includes the use of situations and responses written on 3 x 5 index cards.

Suggested Verbal Presentation

1. The group leader introduces the topic by defining *assertiveness*. The various components of assertion are covered thoroughly in the resources listed in the bibliography. A brief handout is also provided in this exercise, which includes basic definitions of assertion, nonassertion, and aggression.

2. To clarify the differences between assertion, nonassertion, and aggression, the group leader may use the situation and response cards. The leader displays the cards and explains that each set contains a situation and three responses. One group member is asked to read a situation aloud and then three members are each instructed to read a response. Other participants are to indicate whether each response was assertive, aggressive, or nonassertive.

3. Upon completion of each set, the following aspects may be discussed:

a) How was the assertive response different from the others?

b) Which response was the most direct?

c) Which response was an honest expression of feelings?

d) What reactions might you expect to each response?

e) How do the following affect an assertive response: voice tone? facial expressions? body language?

f) Was it difficult to differentiate between the different types of responses?

4. Upon completion of the exercise, the leader summarizes, providing positive feedback for group participation and encourages the participants to become aware of the types of responses they encounter.

DEFINITIONS AND COMPARISONS

The following situations/responses should be written on 3 x 5 cards to be used as a basis for discussion in this exercise.

Situation One:

> You are listening to the stereo and someone changes the record.

Responses:

> 1) You say...*Get your hands off of that stereo. I don't want to listen to your lousy records!* (AGGRESSIVE)
> 2) You leave the room angrily and decide to listen to your portable radio. (NONASSERTIVE)
> 3) You say...*Excuse me, I was listening to that song. If you'd like, you can put on a different record when this one is over.* (ASSERTIVE)

Situation Two:

> You are in a crowded room at a public meeting, sitting next to someone whose cigarette smoke is bothering you.

Responses:

> 1) You angrily sit through the meeting, wishing someone would tell the person to put out the cigarette. (NONASSERTIVE)
> 2) You quietly say...*The smoke from your cigarette is really making me uncomfortable. Would you put your cigarette out?* (ASSERTIVE)
> 3) You loudly tell the person how rude he/she is for not considering the nonsmokers in the room. (AGGRESSIVE)

Situation Three:

> A new friend of yours from work has invited you to a small dinner party. Everyone else at the party seems to know each other quite well.

Responses:

> 1) You quietly listen to the conversation at the dinner table, wishing someone would talk to you. (NONASSERTIVE)

2) You introduce yourself to the person sitting next to you and begin talking about where you met the host or hostesses. (ASSERTIVE)
3) You decide not to be left out and begin to monopolize the conversation, talking about your new job. (AGGRESSIVE)

Situation Four:
Your spouse has decided that he/she wants to spend your week of vacation quietly resting at home but you would rather do some travelling.

Responses:
1) You tell him/her that they are just too cheap and lazy to do anything but lay around all week. (AGGRESSIVE)
2) You decide that he/she works more than you do and needs the rest, even though you really hate the idea of spending your vacation at home. (NONASSERTIVE)
3) You ask your spouse if the vacation plans could be discussed further and suggest a few relaxing but fun places to go for a few days of the vacation. (ASSERTIVE)

ASSERTIVENESS

"Behavior which enables a person to act in his or her own best interests, to stand up for herself or himself without undue anxiety, to express honest feelings comfortably, or to exercise personal rights without denying the rights of others..."*

Nonassertion	Assertion	Aggression

Nonassertion: failing to stand up for oneself, or allowing one's rights to be easily violated.

Aggression: standing up for oneself by violating the rights of another person. Frequently involves putting down the other person.

Alberti RE, Emmons ML: Your Perfect Right, A Guide to Assertive Behavior. San Luis Obispo, California, Impact Pubs, 1978, p 2.

EXERCISE II

Purpose

An opportunity is provided for the group participants to increase awareness of his or her own behaviors in situations which call for assertiveness. This exercise includes the completion of a questionnaire.

Suggested Verbal Presentation

1. The group leader introduces the exercise with the following discussion: *Many people find it easy to be assertive in some situations and very uncomfortable to do so in other situations. How we react frequently depends on the circumstances, particularly upon the relationship with the person involved. Assertive behavior is not universal, therefore, individual differences must be recognized. This exercise will help you to identify the specific areas in which you feel comfortable responding assertively, and those in which you feel less comfortable. There are no right or wrong answers to this questionnaire. It is designed to increase your awareness of your level of comfort in the situation.*

2. The leader distributes the questionnaire to the participants and directs them to complete the exercise. Allow 10 to 15 minutes for the completion of the exercise.

3. After all members have completed the questionnaire, the group leader encourages discussion of the results, considering each item individually. The following discussion questions may be asked:

   a) How did you respond to question one, two, etc...

   b) When a participant replies "sometimes" or any other indefinite answer, ask: *What would make the difference in this situation? When would you feel comfortable? When would you not be comfortable?*

   c) What other situations calling for assertiveness can you identify that would make you feel uncomfortable?

d) With whom are you most comfortable being assertive?

e) With whom are you least comfortable being assertive?

4. After discussing the answers to the questionnaire, the leader summarizes and provides positive feedback for group participation.

Adaptations

1. Several types of "assertiveness inventories" are available in the literature concerning assertiveness training. This abbreviated form has been most successful within a 45 minute time limit.

2. The participants may be given a resource list and encouraged to complete more comprehensive inventories.

ASSERTIVENESS QUESTIONNAIRE

Name: _____

Please answer the following questions honestly and briefly.

1. Do you feel comfortable resisting sales pressure from a salesman? _____
2. Do you feel comfortable returning or exchanging faulty merchandise? _____
3. Do you feel comfortable saying something to someone who has stepped in front of you while waiting in line? _____
4. Do you feel comfortable asking for the return of a borrowed item? _____
5. Do you feel comfortable refusing unreasonable requests from your friends? _____
6. Do you feel comfortable approaching and introducing yourself to a stranger at a party? _____
7. Do you feel comfortable telling your spouse how you feel about something they have done that has hurt you? _____
8. Do you feel comfortable asking others to do a fair share of the work load? _____
9. Do you feel comfortable openly expressing love and affection? _____
10. Do you feel comfortable asking others for help? _____

EXERCISE III

Purpose

The concept of stating needs, rights, and feelings in a direct, assertive manner is focused through the use of role play. This exercise includes the use of situations written on 3 x 5 index cards.

Suggested
Verbal
Presentation

1. The group leader displays the index cards and explains the purpose of the group. The following discussion may be used: *The purpose of this group is to practice stating your feelings and needs in a direct, assertive manner. Each person will select a card, read it aloud, and choose a partner to take the part of the other person involved in the situation. Remember to make your feelings known in an assertive manner.*

2. The group leader asks for a volunteer to select the first card and encourages and supports the role play.

3. After a situation is considered and acted upon, the leader stimulates discussion of the interaction. The following questions may be used to facilitate discussion:

a) What would you be feeling if you were in this situation?

b) Did the person acting out this situation express honest feelings? Were the messages direct?

c) Would anyone have responded differently to this situation?

d) Has anyone been involved in a similar situation?

e) Directed to the actor...Do you feel that you responded assertively?

f) Could you respond assertively if this situation actually occurred to you?

4. Discussion should be encouraged by the group leader of each interaction.

5. After all group participants have an opportunity to role play an assertive response, the leader summarizes, provides positive feedback for group participation, and encourages the members to practice assertive behaviors in their personal-social interactions.

Adaptations

1. Frequently, after two or three situations are role played, group members offer their own situations to be acted upon; therefore, the cards may only be necessary as an "ice breaker."

2. Situations determined by the results of the logsheet in Exercise IV may be used in place of the cards.

3. Card selection may be done at random or may be limited to the category identified by the group leader or participant.

ROLE-PLAY SITUATIONS

The following situations should be written on 3 x 5 index cards if used as a basis for role play in this exercise.

Public

1. You are at a public meeting in a crowded room. A man enters and sits down next to you and lights up an offensive smelling cigar.
2. You are in a restaurant and the waitress has not taken your order. You have been waiting for 40 minutes.

Work

1. There are no problems at work but your supervisor never praises you for your work performance.
2. Your boss is consistantly scheduling you for overtime and it is interfering with your private life.
3. You have started a new job and your boss has given you more responsibility than you can handle comfortably.

Friend

1. You are interested in a date with someone you have recently become acquainted with.
2. You are not busy doing anything, just relaxing. A friend calls and asks you to drive them somewhere for the third time this week.
3. Your friend is always borrowing your clothes and you are getting tired of it.

Relative

1. You have just received a call from your "least favorite" aunt. She is inviting herself to stay with you for a few weeks.
2. One of your relatives is constantly trying to tell you what to do with your life.

Parent

1. You are feeling as if your parent has never treated you like an adult.

2. Your parent has recently been criticizing you about the way you have been dealing with your problems.

Children

1. You are having trouble communicating with your teenage son whom you suspect of using drugs.

2. You are very angry with your children about   (YOU DECIDE)

Spouse

1. Your spouse has been refusing to allow you to be responsible for yourself since your illness.

2. You expected your spouse to be home for dinner right after work. He/she just returned, three hours late, with the explanation that he/she went out for a few drinks with the gang from work.

3. You and your spouse are watching TV and the thought crosses your mind that he/she has not told you that he/she loves you for a long time.

EXERCISE IV

Purpose

An opportunity is provided for the group participants to practice assertive behaviors and to assess the results of the interaction. This exercise includes the completion of a logsheet which may be used as an individual exercise or as an assignment sheet.

**Suggested
Verbal
Presentation**

1. The group leader distributes the worksheet to the group and explains the purpose of the exercise. The following discussion may be used: *This logsheet is to keep a record of the opportunities you have had to be assertive. Keeping such a record will help you to evaluate the situations in which you were assertive and those in which you were not assertive. It will allow you to see your progress in becoming more assertive and may also motivate you to continue practicing assertion.*

2. The leader instructs the group to list two recent situations where they have had the opportunity to be assertive. The situations should be described in Column One. Allow five to seven minutes for the completion of Column One.

3. When the members have completed Column One, the group leader instructs them to indicate whether or not they were assertive. The leader then instructs the group to give the results of their assertion or nonassertion. These results should indicate both the feelings of the participant and the reaction of others involved.

4. Upon completion of the exercise, the group leader encourages discussion through the following questions:

   a) What opportunities to be assertive did you have?

   b) Were you assertive?

   c) How did you feel before you acted? Afterward?

   d) How did the others involved in the situation react?

e) Would you react differently if this situation arose again? In what way?

5. The leader summarizes after all participants have shared their situations and requests that the group members continue to record such situations. Additional logsheets may need to be distributed.

Adaptations

1. The logsheet may be used as an assignment to be discussed at a later discussion group.

Bibliography*

Alberti RE, Emmons ML: Stand Up, Speak Out, Talk Back! New York, Pocket Books, 1975.

Alberti RE, Emmons ML: Your Perfect Right, A Guide To Assertive Behavior. San Luis Obispo, CA, Impact Pub, 1978.

Fensterheim H, Baer J: Don't Say Yes When You Want to Say No. New York, Dell Pub Co Inc, 1975.

Jakubowski-Spector PA: Facilitating the growth of women through assertiveness training. The Counseling Psychologist 4:75-86, 1973.

Lange AJ, Jakubowski PA: Responsible Assertive Behavior: Cognitive Behavioral Procedures For Trainers. Champaign, IL, Research Press, 1976.

Phelps S, Austin N: The Assertive Woman. San Luis Obispo, CA, Impact Pub, 1975.

Smith MJ: When I Say "No" I Feel Guilty. New York, Dial Press, 1975.

Explore community-based Assertiveness Training Programs available in your area.

ASSERTIVENESS LOGSHEET

Name: _____

Situation:	Did You Assert Yourself?	Results:

EMPLOYMENT

Introduction

Occupational therapists often deal with clients who present a broad range of occupational liabilities. These may be on a continuum from those who have never before held a job, to those who have been consistently employed but who tend to deal quite ineffectively with job stresses. This section has been organized to cover the employment scene, including concepts about: 1) self-knowledge as a guide to job choice, 2) preparing for the job market, 3) locating and contacting prospective employers, 4) handling the employment interview, and 5) coping with stress on the job.

Treatment goals include the following:

1. To identify employment interests and resources (EXERCISE I).

2. To identify employment aptitudes and skills (EXERCISES II, III).

3. To identify personality characteristics and relate these to the employment situation (EXERCISE IV).

4. To explore community resources available for gathering job or career information (EXERCISE V).

5. To investigate potential jobs (EXERCISE VI).

6. To match interests, aptitudes, skills, and personality traits with job requirements (EXERCISE VII).

7. To provide an opportunity to complete a sample job application (EXERCISE VIII).

8. To provide an opportunity to learn the purposes and format of a resume and letter of application (EXERCISE IX).

9. To identify expectations for the employment interview through a simulated experience (EXERCISE X).

10. To identify more effective methods of coping with stress on the job (EXERCISES XI, XII).

EXERCISE I

Purpose

Employment interests and resources are identified.

**Suggested
Verbal
Presentation**

1. The leader begins by distributing a copy of the worksheet and introduces the topic with the following discussion: *An important aspect in finding a satisfying job often has to do with your being able to match your interests with the requirements of the job. For example, an individual who likes working with his hands might find a job as a tool-and-die maker more satisfying than, say, if he were a salesman. There are many factors that contribute to making a particular job satisfying for an individual. This exercise is designed to help you identify some preferences. Establishing your likes and dislikes can serve as a useful guide for the jobs you later seek.*

2. The leader directs the group to look at the worksheet. The group is to circle "a" or "b," whichever is preferred. Allow approximately ten minutes for completion of the exercise.

3. When everyone has finished, the leader promotes discussion about the outcome of the exercise. This could be accomplished by having individuals verbally indicate to the group their responses or by having the group as a whole indicate by show of hands their responses to the various statements. Discussion questions might include:

 a) Why did you prefer this choice over the other one?

 b) Do you have any ideas about the kinds of jobs that might match your interests? How could you obtain more information about this?

 c) What are some of the other factors that should be considered when looking for a job?

4. The leader summarizes, providing positive feedback for group participation and reiterating the main points of the topic.

Adaptations

1. If the group has verbal or visual limitations, the leader may want to read through each section.

2. The worksheet can be modified by selecting, for example, ten statements from the worksheet. These could be listed on another worksheet or on the blackboard. The group is then directed to indicate their three main interests. This type of modification has been helpful with lower-functioning groups.

INTERESTS AND RESOURCES

Name: _____

Which Do You Prefer? (Circle "a" or "b")

1. (a) Making decisions   (b) Having decisions made for you

2. (a) Motivating others   (b) Having others motivate you

3. (a) Directing and supervising others   (b) Being supervised and directed by someone

4. (a) Competing with others   (b) Being in a situation in which there is little or competition among people

5. (a) Solving problems   (b) Having problems explained to you

6. (a) Working with people   (b) Working with things

7. (a) Working independently   (b) Working as part of a team

8. (a) Working with detail, ie, numbers or technical written material   (b) Helping people

9. (a) Following step-by-step directions   (b) Creating a project

9. (a) Following step-by-step directions   (b) Creating a project from your own ideas

10. (a) Working inside   (b) Working outside

EXERCISE II

Purpose

Employment aptitudes and skills are identified.

Suggested
Verbal
Presentation

1. The leader distributes a copy of the worksheet and begins with the following discussion: *The purpose of this exercise is to have you take a look at the kind of person you are. By being more aware of your likes, dislikes, accomplishments, failures, interests, and disinterests, you become more in touch with your personal needs and wants. This can be quite helpful when you are trying to make a decision about the type of job to pursue. In completing the exercise, address yourself to the questions listed at the top of the sheet.*

2. The leader directs the group to take approximately 20 minutes for completion of the exercise.

3. When everyone has finished, the leader encourages participants to share their findings. Since time may be a factor, it may be more productive to have participants briefly summarize what they wrote. Another way to approach this is to ask some of the specific questions indicated at the top of the worksheet, encouraging each participant to respond, ie, *What have been some of your accomplishments?*

4. When each has had an opportunity to focus in on the key areas, the leader summarizes.

Adaptations

1. Sometimes it may be necessary to do this exercise in two sessions: the first session is used to explain the exercise and allow sufficient time to respond more thoroughly to each question; the second session is used mainly for discussion and feedback.

2. The exercise can be given as an assignment that participants complete over a period of a few days, at times convenient to them. The deadline is set as the next group meeting time.

APTITUDES AND SKILLS

Name: _____

What Kind of Person Are You?
What Are Your Interests?
What Are Your Accomplishments?
What Has Given You Satisfaction in the Past?
What Has Made You Unhappy?

In the space below, write a brief autobiography. The purpose is to set down and review all the components that have interacted to produce the kind of individual you are.

_____

_____

_____

_____

_____

_____

_____

_____

_____

_____

_____

_____

_____

_____

EXERCISE III

Purpose

Employment aptitudes and skills are identified.

Suggested
Verbal
Presentation

1. The leader distributes a copy of the worksheet and begins with the following discussion: *In this exercise we want you to identify what you personally consider some of your strengths and weaknesses. Your assets are your personal resources that you can utilize in different situations. They are your strengths, either natural personality traits or developed skills. While assets are often more appealing to consider, you can learn much about yourself by taking a good look at your shortcomings. These can serve as a guide and being aware of them can often be as helpful to you as your assets are. Having identified some shortcomings, you may decide these are areas you want to work on to improve.*

2. The leader directs the group to look at the worksheet. A brief explanation may be necessary. Avoid prompting the group by giving suggestions as to responses that could be made (often you will find that these are the ones that appear). Allow 15 minutes for completion.

3. When everyone has finished, the leader encourages participants to share their ideas. The leader may want to have participants share their descriptive word first, then individually state assets/shortcomings.

4. The leader summarizes, providing positive feedback for group participation and reiterating the main points of the topic.

Adaptations

1. Lengthen or shorten the number of assets or shortcomings that participants should indicate.

APTITUDES AND SKILLS

Name: _____

Describe Yourself in One Word:

```
┌─────────────────────┐
│                     │
│                     │
└─────────────────────┘
```

List Five Assets:	List Five Shortcomings:
1 _____	1 _____
_____	_____
2 _____	2 _____
_____	_____
3 _____	3 _____
_____	_____
4 _____	4 _____
_____	_____
5 _____	5 _____
_____	_____

EXERCISE IV

Purpose

Personality characteristics are identified. These can be incorporated into a discussion of the types of jobs an individual is considering. It can also be beneficial to use in conjunction with the exercise dealing with job stresses to provide the leader and the participant with an indication of the participant's self-concept. A pattern of responses in the left-hand column indicate a relatively positive self-concept; a pattern of responses in the right-hand column indicate a rather negative self-concept.

Suggested Verbal Presentation

1. The leader distributes a copy of the worksheet and directs the group to respond to the question: *how would you describe yourself?* There are two adjectives on each line, separated by five circles. Responses are made by darkening in the circle that a person feels best describes himself. For example, someone may respond to the statement:

OPTIMISTIC o-o-o-●-o PESSIMISTIC

This may indicate that he generally feels pessimistic, but does not always feel that way.

2. When the leader is confident that everyone understands the exercise, the group is directed to take about 15 minutes to complete the worksheet.

3. When everyone is finished, the leader asks the group members if they are interested in getting feedback about their responses. This part of the exercise has proved particularly sensitive in some cases, and it is recommended it be done only if the participants are interested in comparing their self-evaluations with how different group members view them. If participants are interested in the feedback, encourage them to choose those group members they would prefer getting feedback from. "Inflicting" group members on

each other may provoke uncalled for hostilities. The leader should point out that group members evaluating each other should try to remain objective. The partners simply check *agree* or *disagree* next to each statement. After each assessment, it is most productive to have the partners individually discuss their responses with each other for clarification.

4. The leader promotes discussion about group member's feelings about the exercise and explains to the group the positive and negative response patterns. This may be obvious to some of the group, but an explanation often facilitates discussion with group members disagreeing with the explanation.

5. The leader may want to focus the discussion on areas such as:

a) How does your self-evaluation compare with your partner's views of you?

b) How did you and your partner handle disagreements? How did you each feel?

c) How do other people form impressions of us? In what ways do we communicate who we are, what we feel, what we like, etc?

6. The leader summarizes, encouraging participants to repeat the exercise at some time in the future to see if their views of themselves have undergone any changes.

Adaptations

1. This exercise can be done at the time of admission or initial contact with a client and redone at later stages of progress as an assessment of improved self-concept.

PERSONALITY CHARACTERISTICS

Name: _____

	Partner #1		Partner #2	
	Agree	Disagree	Agree	Disagree
Intelligent o-o-o-o Less Intelligent				
Extrovert o-o-o-o Introvert				
Adventuresome o-o-o-o Timid				
Confident o-o-o-o Unsure				
Loving o-o-o-o Hostile				
Trusting o-o-o-o Cautious				
Carefree o-o-o-o Worrying				
Sensitive o-o-o-o Insensitive				
Ambitious o-o-o-o Not ambitious				
Honest o-o-o-o Dishonest				
Generous o-o-o-o Frugal				
Optimistic o-o-o-o Pessimistic				
Realistic o-o-o-o Idealistic				
Sense of Humor o-o-o-o Humorless				
Independent o-o-o-o Dependent				
Courageous o-o-o-o Not Courageous				
Conscientious o-o-o-o Irresponsible				
Open-minded o-o-o-o Opinionated				
Practical o-o-o-o Impractical				
Passionate o-o-o-o Cool				

EXERCISE V

Purpose

    Community resources available for gathering job or career information are explored. This exercise relies heavily on the leader to present each area listed on the handout and to promote group discussion surrounding previous use of the different resources and the outcomes.

**Suggested
Verbal
Presentation**

    1. The leader distributes a copy of the handout and begins with the following discussion: *We are going to take a look at some of the resources you have available to you when you go to look for a job. Some of these you may have used before and some you may not be familiar with. As we discuss each area, please share with the group any experiences you have had that are related and indicate whether it was relatively helpful or not to you.*

    a) Want Ads: The leader may want to take a copy of the classified section of the local newspaper to the group, with one or two advertisements circled in red. Encourage a volunteer to read an advertisement and have the group focus on the information.

    b) Personal Friends: Employed friends may be aware of job openings where they work.

    c) Private Employment Agencies: These agencies generally advertise their services in the classified section of the newspaper and are often listed in the telephone directory. The employer sometimes but not always pays the fee for locating an individual in a job. Agreements must be understood before they are signed. Be sure the agency is reputable.

    d) State Employment Office: They often have listings regarding available civil service job openings as well as jobs listed by private companies.

101

e) High School Counseling Office: Companies some-times list temporary or part-time positions with these offices. The can assist with career planning.

f) College Placement Office: This can be a useful source of job openings for individuals with special training.

g) Civil Service Office: A civil service office lists positions available, including special training or test score requirements.

h) Directories: Directories are generally available at local libraries. They can be a good source of jobs because companies often have openings but do not advertise. The individual should take the initiative to send a resume.

i) Department of Vocational Rehabilitation: It should be emphasized to the group that this agency should be utilized by individuals who meet the qualifications for the service, as defined in your area. An explanation of the procedure utilized in your facility to refer candidates to this agency and a description of the way in which the agency functions can be beneficial to the participants.

2. Some discussion questions may include:

a) Who has used this kind of service?

b) What were the results?

c) Would you consider using this service again?

d) What were some of the problems associated with using this service?

e) Can you describe more specifically how you went about using this resource?

3. The leader summarizes, providing positive feedback for group participation and reiterating the main points of the discussion.

COMMUNITY RESOURCES

Where Can I Find Out About Job Openings..........?

Want Ads
Personal Friends
Private Employment Agencies
State Employment Office
High School Counseling Office
College Placement Office
Civil Service Office
Directories: Telephone Book
             Chamber of Commerce Lists
             Membership Rosters of Trade
               and Professional Organizations
Department of Vocational Rehabilitation

EXERCISE VI

Purpose

Potential jobs are investigated.

Suggested
Verbal
Presentation

1. The leader distributes a copy of the worksheet, briefly explains the format and provides directions for completion of it, and makes the group aware of the resources available to them to complete the exercise. Suggested reference materials include the following: *The Occupational Outlook Handbook; The Dictionary of Occupational Titles;* and newspaper want ads.

2. The leader directs the group to share the materials and to work together as much as possible to complete their worksheets. Allow approximately 20 to 25 minutes for completion of the worksheets.

3. When everyone has finished, the leader promotes discussion about the outcome of the exercise. This can be accomplished by encouraging participants to share the information they gathered. Possible discussion questions include:

a) Why did you choose this job?

b) What was your main resource for gathering the information on it?

c) Were any group members able to provide you with additional information? If so, who?

d) Were the resources here adequate to gather all the necessary information?

e) If you wanted to use these resources in the future, where might you find them?

4. The leader summarizes, providing positive feedback for group participation and reiterating the main points of the topic.

Adaptations

1. This exercise can be assigned as an individual task to be completed on a client's own time outside of the group. Then results can be shared during the formal group discussion.

INVESTIGATING POTENTIAL JOBS

Name: _____

Using the *Occupational Outlook Handbook*, the
Dictionary of Occupational Titles, or some other
available resource (book, newspaper, etc)
investigate three jobs of interest to you.

	Job Title	Where Employed	Duties	Training or Experience Needed	Pay
Job #1					
Job #2					
Job #3					

EXERCISE VII

Purpose

Interests, aptitudes, skills, and personality are matched with job requirements. This exercise is most beneficial if utilized after group members have completed exercises I, II, III, and IV. Although it is not absolutely essential, it helps in promoting discussion about the relationship between the above areas if participants are more acutely aware of their individual needs and wants. Therefore, at least one of the self-exploration exercises is recommended prior to completion of this one.

Suggested Verbal Presentation

1. The leader distributes a copy of the worksheet and begins with the following explanation: *In this exercise, we are going to take a look at your specific employment interests. First, fold the sheet along the dotted lines and begin by listing five jobs that you would definitely want to be working at. Be sure to indicate why in the space to the right of each response.* Allow about 10 minutes for completion of this part.

2. When everyone has completed the first part, the leader instructs the group to complete the second part in the same manner. Allow 10 minutes for completion of this part.

3. At this point the leader may want to distribute to the participants any of the self-evaluation exercise materials they completed at an earlier time. This will greatly facilitate discussion about the relationship between personal criteria with employment requirements/responsibilities.

4. The leader promotes discussion by encouraging group members to share their responses to the worksheet. Suggested discussion questions include:

a) What were the main personality traits you identified in the earlier exercise?

b) What were some of the jobs you preferred? clearly disliked?

c) Do you see any relationship between the jobs you seemed to prefer with some of your personal qualities? What do others think?

d) What were some of the reasons you gave for the jobs you disliked?

e) Do others have any ideas what types of jobs might fit in with the ones (John) indicated he preferred?

5. The leader summarizes, providing positive feedback for group participation and reiterating the main points of the discussion.

Adaptations

1. Lengthen or shorten the number of jobs to be indicated.

MATCHING YOU WITH YOUR JOB

Name: _____

**List Five Jobs that
Appeal to You:**   **Why?**

1. _____   _____

2. _____   _____

3. _____   _____

4. _____   _____

5. _____   _____

— — — — — — — — — — — — — — — — — — — —

**List Five Jobs that
Definitely Do Not
Appeal to You:**   **Why?**

1. _____   _____

2. _____   _____

3. _____   _____

4. _____   _____

5. _____   _____

EXERCISE VIII

Purpose

> To provide an opportunity to complete a sample job application.

**Suggested
Verbal
Presentation**

> 1. The leader distributes a copy of the worksheet and begins with the following discussion: *The purpose of this exercise is to give you an opportunity to complete a sample job application. It will give you an idea of the kinds of information an employer is interested in. We will go through each section together, with you filling in the information. If at any time you do not understand, please ask questions.*
>
> 2. The leader reads each section and the participants fill in the appropriate information. Clarify any questions that arise. Most of the discussion should occur during completion of each section. Encourage the group to make their own decisions about responses to the different sections; it is good to encourage discussion about the pros and cons of various responses.
>
> 3. When the group has finished, the leader summarizes, reiterating some of the main points of the discussion.

Adaptations

> An individual may feel more comfortable completing this at his leisure and discussing it later.

Position Applied For _____

Date _____

Name _____ Last First Middle

Social Sec.# _____

Address _____ Street City State Zip Code

Citizen of United States ☐ Yes ☐ No   If not, type of Visa _____

Education

Highest Level of Schooling (Check One)	If College, Major Field of Study	List Schools Attended	Location	Years Attended	Year Graduated
☐ 0. Less than high school ☐ 1. High School of G.E.D. ☐ 2. College, no degree ☐ 3. Associate Degree ☐ 4. Bachelors ☐ 5. Masters ☐ 6. Doctorate	☐ 0. Not Applicable ☐ 1. Business ☐ 2. Social Science ☐ 3. Biological ☐ 4. Pure Science ☐ 5. Paramedical ☐ 6. Liberal Arts ☐ 7. Education ☐ 8. Other	High School Business or Trade School College College			

EXPLOYMENT EXPERIENCE (Start with your most recent job and work back.)

EMPLOYER	ADDRESS	YOUR POSITION	DATES	REASON FOR LEAVING

Have you ever been convicted for other than a minor traffic violation ☐ Yes ☐ No

I certify that all statements are true and any misrepresentation may cause my separation. I authorize investigation of all statements here.

_____
Signature

111

EXERCISE IX

Purpose

To provide an opportunity to learn the purposes
and format of a resume and letter of application.

Suggested Verbal Presentation

1. The leader distributes a copy of each handout ("Guidelines for the Application Letter" and "Resume Format") and begins with the following discussion: *The purpose of this exercise is to give you an opportunity to learn how to write an application letter and resume. First, let's look at the way in which each of these is used. We will start by closely examining the content of the application letter.*

2. The leader encourages a participant to read from the application letter handout. Clarify each section as it is read.

3. When the content of the application letter has been fully discussed, the leader might encourage the participants to practice writing their own letters. These could be discussed at a later group.

4. The leader now directs the group's attention to the resume format and reviews the content. Clarify any questions the participants may have.

5. When all content areas of the resume format have been clarified, the leader might want to encourage the participants to compile their own resumes, which could be discussed at a later group.

6. The leader summarizes, reiterating the main points of the exercise.

Adaptations

1. This exercise can be divided into two separate sessions:

Session I: Review the application letter format and have the group compile their individual letters during group time. Use the group as a "work session." Have each participant read their letter to the group and provide feedback as to content, clarity, etc.

Session II: Review the resume format and have the group compile their individual resumes during the group time ("work session" as above). Evaluate each resume as was done with the application letter and provide feedback to the participant.

GUIDELINES FOR THE APPLICATION LETTER

Your Return Address
Street, City, State, Zip Code
Today's Date

Person To Whom You Are Sending This Letter
Company's Name
Company's Address

Dear _____ :

(Opening Paragraph): Introduce yourself and provide some brief information about your background or skills. Indicate the kind of position in which you are interested. Be specific.

(Body of Letter): Indicate some of the reasons you are interested in a position with this particular company. Provide information about prior work experience, special talents, and accomplishments as they relate to the specific position for which you are applying. If you are including a resume, draw the reader's attention to this.

(Final Paragraph): Express your interest in a personal interview, and indicate your flexibility as to date and time.

Sincerely,

Your Name
Your Telephone Number

RESUME FORMAT

Your name
Address
Telephone Number

Position Desired:

Personal:	Date of Birth	Health
	Height	Military Status
	Weight	Marital Status

Education:
    High School: Name, Address
    College: Name, Address, Major, Minor, Degree

Work Experience: (Start with most recent and work back.)
1. Name of Company
   Responsibilities
   Reason for Leaving

2. Name of Company
   Responsibilities
   Reasons for Leaving

References:
1. Name
   Position
   Address

2. Name
   Position
   Address

EXERCISE X

Purpose

Expectations for the employment interview and a simulated experience are provided.

Suggested
Verbal
Presentation

1. The leader distributes a copy of each handout ("Guidelines
for the Employment Interview" and "Some Questions to
Anticipate During the Employment Interview") and begins
with the following discussion: *In this exercise we will review
some guidelines for the employment interview and take a
look at questions you might expect to be asked during the
interview. At the end of the discussion, you will have an
opportunity to practice an interview.*

2. The leader directs the group's attention to the handout,
"Guidelines for the Employment Interview." As each section
is read, the leader can assess the group's understanding of it
by asking participants to explain more fully and in their own
words the content of each point. This approach also
facilitates group interaction and decreases the chances of the
format becoming a lecture presentation by the leader.

3. The leader now directs the group's attention to the
handout, "Some Questions To Anticipate During the
Employment Interview." The group can be divided into
dyads, with one member acting as the interviewer and the
other the person being interviewed. The group is to follow the
questions presented on the handout. The roles are then
reversed.

4. When the group has completed this part of the exercise,
the leader facilitates group discussion about the outcome of
the experience. Some discussion questions might include:

a) How did you feel during the interview?

b) Do you think you did a good job? What areas do you
think you might improve on?

c) What does your "partner" think about your performance? Do you agree/disagree?

d) Did you remember to follow the guidelines we discussed at the beginning of the group?

5. The leader summarizes, providing positive feedback for group participation and reiterating the main points of the discussion.

Adaptations

1. The leader may want to divide this exercise into two separate sessions, particularly if the group is lower-functioning.

GUIDELINES FOR THE EMPLOYMENT INTERVIEW

1. Personal appearance is important. You should dress neatly, appropriately, and be well-groomed.
2. Be punctual. It is better to arrive somewhat early than to rush in at the last minute.
3. Go to the interview prepared to answer questions similar to those on the handout, "Questions to Anticipate."
4. Be courteous and polite.
5. Let the interviewer lead with the questions.
6. Listen attentively to all questions. If you do not understand what is being asked, be sure to seek clarification.
7. Respond honestly to all questions.
8. Be aware of your body language during the interview.
9. When the interviewer has finished asking you questions, you usually will have an opportunity to ask some questions of your own. Asking questions demonstrates a real interest in the position.
10. Avoid negative comments about present or past work situations.

SOME QUESTIONS TO ANTICIPATE DURING THE EMPLOYMENT INTERVIEW

1. Have you applied for positions with companies other than this one?
2. What aspects of your background experience make you particularly qualified for this position?
3. Why did you leave your last job?
4. What do you look for in a job?
5. Are you willing to work overtime or weekends?
6. What kind of people do you get along with best?
7. How have you felt about previous bosses or supervisors? Co-workers? Subordinates?
8. List some of your strong points. List some of your weak points.
9. List some of your short-term goals. List some of your long-term goals.
10. What are your interests outside of work?

EXERCISE XI

Purpose

To identify more effective methods of coping with stress on the job.

Suggested
Verbal
Presentation

1. The leader displays the situation cards explaining that the cards include a number of situations which often occur on the job. The leader points out that each person will select a card, read the situation aloud, and then attempt to explain how they might handle that particular situation.

2. The leader asks for a volunteer to try the first card. Discussion could be encouraged through the use of the following questions:

a) How would you react if this happened to you?

b) Would anyone handle this situation in a different manner?

c) How would you feel if this happened to you?

d) Would you feel competent in your ability to handle this situation?

3. Proceed with the situations until the time limit is reached.

4. The leader summarizes, reiterating some of the main points that were discussed.

Adaptations

1. Situations can be added which are relevant to the group; inappropriate situations can be deleted.

2. Several small discussion groups could be formed to discuss four to five situations each and then present their ideas to the larger group.

3. The situations can be done in a role-play format.

4. An exercise could be formed with the purpose of identifying situations for future group use.

COPING WITH JOB STRESS

The following may be written out on 3 x 5 index cards and distributed individually for discussion.

How Would You Handle The Following Situations?

1. Your supervisor is closely supervising your work.
2. A co-worker often makes rude remarks to you.
3. You feel you are being overworked.
4. Your supervisor has given you a task to do and you do not think you can handle it.
5. You are having trouble getting up in the morning and being on time for work.
6. You are bored with your job.
7. Your boss often gives you last minute jobs that he wants done "right away."
8. You are experiencing many personal problems at home and cannot seem to keep your mind on your work.
9. Your supervisor criticizes you because he feels you did a poor job with your last assignment.
10. You are praised for a job well-done.
11. Co-workers ignore suggestions you make.
12. It is your first day on a job and everything seems to be going wrong.
13. You deal with the public every day. An irate customer is making abusive remarks at you.
14. You have made plans for the evening. Your boss insists you work overtime to complete an assignment.
15. Your boss makes a pass at you.
16. A co-worker has been given credit for your work.
17. Your boss criticizes you in front of your co-workers.
18. You feel you deserve a raise.

EXERCISE XII

Purpose

To identify more effective methods of coping with stress on the job. This is accomplished by having participants examine areas of concern to them personally, their general response to these, and the outcome of the situation.

Suggested Verbal Presentation

1. The leader distributes a copy of the worksheet and begins with the following discussion: *In this exercise we want you to examine your own job situation and identify two things that really bother you. These are to be indicated in the space provided. Next, consider how you generally respond to the situation. Last of all, indicate what you feel is the outcome to your reaction.* Allow 10 to 15 minutes for completion of this part.

2. When the group has finished, the leader promotes discussion. Some questions might include:

   a) What things really bother you at work?

   b) How do you handle each of these?

   c) What generally is the outcome?

   d) How would other people handle the situation?

   e) What might be the outcome to that way of handling it?

   f) Has anyone else experienced the same kind of problem on their job?

   g) How did you handle it? What was the outcome?

Adaptations

1. As the group discusses each person's method of handling different situations, the leader may encourage the participants to indicate any reasonable alternative methods on the reverse side of the paper.

JOB STRESS

Identify Two Things That Really Bother You At Work

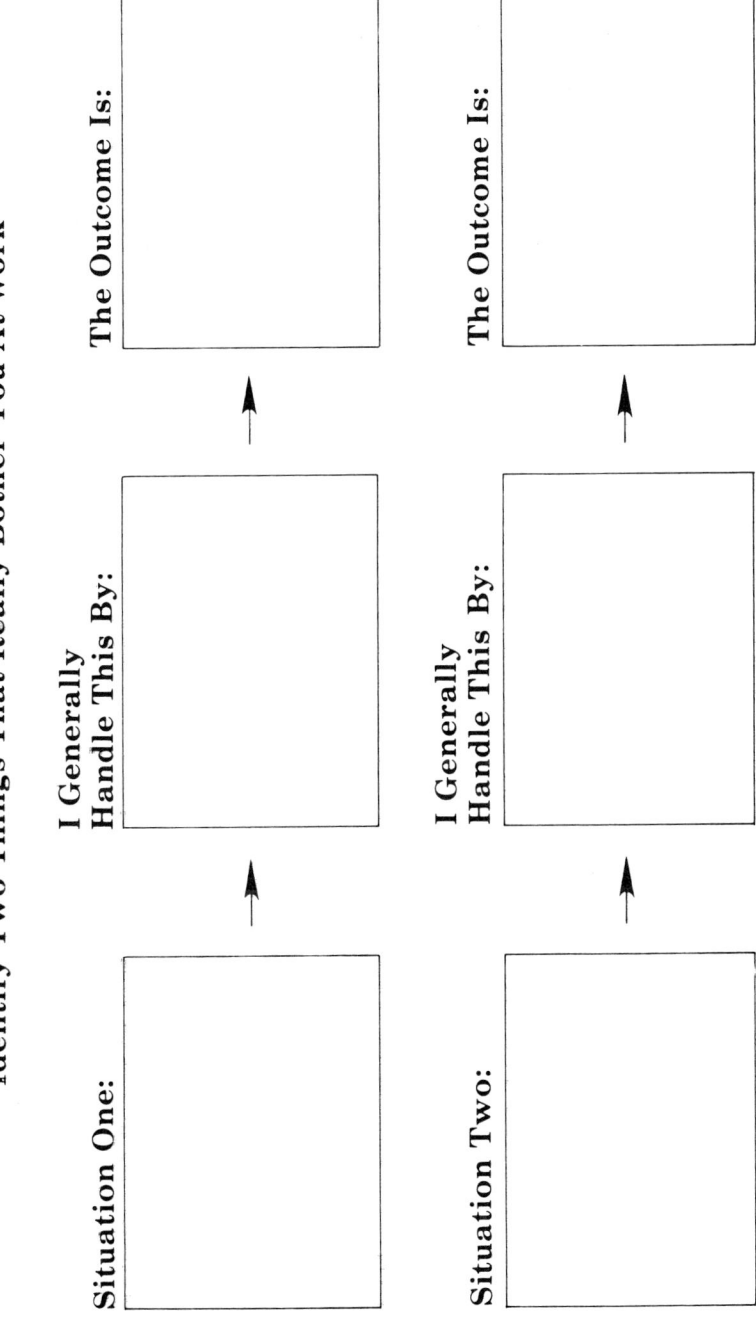

Situation One:

I Generally
Handle This By:

The Outcome Is:

Situation Two:

I Generally
Handle This By:

The Outcome Is:

Bibliography

Barnewall G: Succeed As A Job Applicant. New York, Arco Pub Co, 1977.

Bostwick B: Finding The Job You've Always Wanted. New York, John Wiley & Sons, 1977.

Fear R: The Evaluation Interview, ed 2. New York, McGraw-Hill Book Co, 1973.

Levitan S, Magnum G, Marshall R: Human Resources And Labor Markets, Labor And Manpower In The American Economy. New York, Harper & Row Pubs, 1972.

US Department of Labor, Bureau of Labor Statistics: The Occupational Outlook Handbook. Washington, DC, US Government Printing Office, 1978-79.

US Department of Labor, Employment and Training Administration: The Dictionary of Occupational Titles, ed 4. Washington, DC, US Government Printing Office, 1977.

MONEY MANAGEMENT

Introduction

This section has been organized to assist the occupational therapist who is interested in developing money management skills in clients who demonstrate this need. It consists of a series of discussion groups with specific exercises designed to stimulate learning in this area. As consumers, clients often need to develop problem-solving techniques useful to their particular economic and sociocultural situation. Managing money successfully is a complex skill and is one that is important for independent functioning.

The authors have experienced considerable reluctance on the part of many clients to discuss their financial problems, particularly in group situations. Often, these same clients are receptive to identifying problem areas and looking at alternatives on an individual basis with the therapist, or if the material is presented in general terms rather than dealing with specific issues of a personal nature.

Treatment goals include the following:

1. To explore and identify values and priorities (EXERCISE I).

2. To develop an awareness of spending habits (EXERCISE II).

3. To develop money management plans: setting short- and long-term goals. (EXERCISE III).

4. To identify expenses and compare these with income and goals. (EXERCISE IV).

5. To provide information about establishing a budget. (EXERCISE V).

6. Functioning as a knowledgeable consumer: a look at resources and requirements. (EXERCISE VI).

EXERCISE I

Purpose

      Priorities and values are identified.

Suggested
Verbal
Presentation

      1. The leader begins with the following discussion: *Each person's values affect what he or she spends their money on. Those items that are very important to me may be meaningless to the next person. This exercise is designed to make each of you more aware of what your values are.*

      2. The leader distributes the worksheet and continues with these instructions: *Consider your spending pattern over the past five years. Now look at the worksheet. We will be rating the four areas in terms of their priority to us. It is important to read through each area before assigning a priority to it.*

      3. After the worksheet is read, the group is directed to indicate priorities, with "one" being the greatest priority. Allow approximately five minutes for completion of this part.

      4. When the group has finished, the leader encourages discussion, possibly by exploring examples of items purchased, relevance to individual, or family wants or needs, etc.

      5. The leader summarizes, providing positive feedback for group participation and reiterating the main points of the topic.

Adaptations

      1. Instead of utilizing the worksheet provided, the leader may begin by having the group identify purchases over the past few years. When this is done, the leader may present the four categories and direct the group to categorize their purchases under the appropriate heading. Higher functioning groups have responded better to this approach.

VALUES AND PRIORITIES

Name _____

Shopping Values: Rate the following areas 1, 2, 3, 4, with #1 being your greatest priority:

Self-Improvement

Money Spent on Looking Attractive, Developing Abilities and Interests, and Being Physically Fit.

Family Life

Money Spent on Family Activities and Entertainment, Making Your Home Comfortable and Pleasant.

Special Interests

Money Spent on Musical Instruments, Sports Equipment, Lessons, and Events Related to Talents and Interests.

Knowledge

Money Spent on Education, Books, School Supplies, Tuition and Fees, Savings to Pay College Costs.

EXERCISE II

Purpose

An awareness of spending habits is developed.

Suggested
Verbal
Presentation

1. The leader distributes the worksheet and begins with the following discussion: *This exercise is designed to help you become more aware of your spending habits. Because personal values can differ to a great extent, your particular style of spending money may be very satisfying for you. Check "a," "b," or "c," whichever applies to you.*

2. The leader directs the group to take approximately 15 minutes for completion of this part.

3. When the group is finished, the leader directs the group to place totals in the spaces provided.

4. The leader provides a description of each style, using the following guidelines:

a) *The "a" responses tend to be indicative of the conservative spending style. This pattern often ensures financial security but restricts many of life's satisfactions. A financial plan that includes short- and long-term goals may help to provide a better balance between security and satisfaction.*

b) *The "c" responses tend to represent an impulsive spending style. Since this style often lacks planning, the tendency is to spend more than one has. There is the possibility of eventually getting into substantial debt. Long-term goals and needs may be sacrificed for more immediate desires. Developing a financial plan may provide more realistic management of finances.*

c) *'The "b" responses reflect a moderate spending style. There is a good balance between financial responsibilities and satisfactions. A plan of short- and long-term goals may improve the situation even further.*

5. The leader encourages discussion about the outcome of the exercise, assessing agreement or disagreement with each individual's personal views of themselves.

6. The leader summarizes, providing positive feedback for group participation and reiterating the main points of the topic.

Adaptations

1. The leader may want to read each section aloud, particularly if the group has verbal or visual limitations.

SPENDING HABITS†

Name: _____

(Mark a, b, or c, whichever applies to you.)

_____ 1. (a) I make a purchase only after careful consideration.
      (b) If I buy something spontaneously, I know where the money is coming from.
      (c) I buy something whenever I feel like it.

_____ 2. (a) I seldom spend money on pleasure or entertainment.
      (b) Entertainment is important to me and I plan for it in my budget.
      (c) I spend money on entertainment whenever I feel like it.

_____ 3. (a) I spend considerably less than I have to and save the rest.
      (b) I spend my money on necessities, some luxuries, and put some into savings.
      (c) I generally overspend and have nothing left to save.

_____ 4. (a) I can tell you where every penny is spent.
      (b) I know what my monthly expenses are and plan for them in my budget.
      (c) Some months I have no idea what my expenses will be.

_____ 5. (a) I spend my money only on absolutely essential items.
      (b) I know what I value and I spend my money on the most important things.
      (c) I find I often buy things that I get tired of quickly.

---

†*Adapted with permission from a circular printed and distributed by Manufacturer's Bank, entitled "Money Planner."*

_____6. If I am purchasing a major item (car, appliance, etc):
   (a) I take a long time and shop very carefully for the best buy.
   (b) I set up a reasonable plan, then shop and compare prices for the best value.
   (c) I just buy it and avoid alot of time spent shopping around.

_____7. (a) I never or rarely make credit purchases.
   (b) I plan credit purchases within my budget and make the payments comfortably.
   (c) I often overextend my credit and have difficulty making the payments.

_____8. If confronted with a financial emergency today:
   (a) I could definitely handle it. I plan on emergencies.
   (b) I could handle it with some savings or be able to get additional money.
   (c) I probably could not handle it.

_____9. When purchasing a minor item:
   (a) I debate whether or not I really need it.
   (b) I know it can fit into my overall budget.
   (c) I just buy it without much thought.

****

TOTAL "a"s_____   TOTAL "b"s_____

TOTAL "c"s_____

EXERCISE III

Purpose

Financial plans are developed by identifying short- and long-term goals.

Suggested
Verbal
Presentation

1. The leader distributes the worksheet and begins by explaining: *Goals serve as a guide to spending. In order to set goals, it is necessary to be aware of the things that are important to you and your family.*

2. The leader directs the group's attention to the worksheet and has the group fold the sheet along the dotted lines. Part One is to be completed first. Allow ten minutes for this to be done.

3. When the group has finished, the leader instructs the group to open the worksheet and indicate which items are more important for the short- and long-term. Allow ten minutes for completion of this part.

4. When the group has finished, the leader promotes discussion. Discussion questions might include:

   a) What were two of your short-term goals? (long?)

   b) Are these realistic in terms of your income and expenses?

   c) Do you think your spouse/family would agree or disagree with you? Can you be specific?

   d) How might you reach some of these goals?

   e) Can you sit down with your family and establish some goals together?

5. The leader summarizes, providing positive feedback for group participation and reiterating the main points of the discussion. The summary statement might include the following: *Once you have identified personal and family goals, you can plan the use of your time, money, energy, and ability to reach these. Goals will help you make sound buying decisions.*

132

Adaptations

1. Have the group attempt an estimate of cost for various items indicated.

2. Limit the number of items the group can indicate in Part One.

3. Make an assignment for group members to actually sit down with their families and do the exercise together.

4. The therapist might sit down with a client and the family to complete the exercise.

5. The exercise can be done in two separate groups if time must be limited or the therapist is dealing with a lower functioning group.

SHORT AND LONG-TERM GOALS

Name: _____

Financial Goals: Write down all the things you want that money can buy.

_____

Important To Me Now: | **Important For The Future:**

EXERCISE IV

Purpose

Monthly expenses are identified and expenses are compared with income. Ways of achieving short- and long-term goals are explored.

Suggested
Verbal
Presentation

1. The leader distributes the worksheet and begins by explaining the purpose of the exercise.

2. The group is instructed to indicate on the worksheet as many monthly expenses as they are normally confronted with and to approximate the amount in the column to the right. Allow ten minutes for completion of this part.

3. When the group has finished, the leader directs the group to total their expenses, writing this in the space provided, and to indicate their monthly income.

4. The leader promotes discussion through questions such as:

a) Do you live within your income?

b) What are particular problem areas? (Some areas that the group defines in this section might be useful to include in Exercise VI.)

c) Which expenses might be cut down somewhat?

d) Are you able to meet any short- or long-term goals with your present spending pattern? If yes, how? If no, why? Can this be changed?

5. The leader summarizes, providing positive feedback for group participation and reiterating the main points of the discussion.

Adaptations

1. The purpose of having the group members indicate their

expenses without the assistance of a complete listing of expenses is to give the leader an opportunity to assess individual awareness of finances. If the group is lower functioning or time is a problem, the leader may want to initially present a composite list on the blackboard and have the group use this as a guide. A suggested list might include:

rent or payment
electricity
telephone
heating
taxes
water
food
car: gas/oil
         repairs
insurance:
         life
         car
         health
loan payments

allowances
medical expenses
cleaning/laundry
tuition
other educational expenses
church donations
other donations
entertainment
babysitter
dues
savings
alimony/support payments
house/appliance repairs

IDENTIFYING EXPENSES

Name: _____

List Your Expenses and the Approximate Amount

Item	Amount
_____	_____
_____	_____
_____	_____
_____	_____
_____	_____
_____	_____
_____	_____
_____	_____
_____	_____
_____	_____
_____	_____
_____	_____
_____	_____

Total _____

Total Income   _____
Total Expenses _____
                _____

Some Possible Expenses

Rent or Payment
Electricity
Telephone
Heating
Water
Food
Car: Gas/oil
       Repairs
       Insurance
Barber/Beauty Shop

Loan Payments
Allowances
Health Insurance
Cleaning-Laundry
Tuition
Church Donations
Entertainment
Babysitter
Savings

EXERCISE V

Purpose

Some basic information is introduced about establishing a budget. This exercise should be used after the group has completed Exercise IV.

Suggested
Verbal
Presentation

1. The leader distributes the worksheet and begins with the following discussion: *A budget is a plan that allows you to coordinate your resources and your expenses. Within your budget, you decide how much money is available for or required for a particular purpose. An important aspect of setting up a budget is identifying which expenses are "fixed" and which are "flexible." A fixed expense never varies, or rarely does so. An example of this might be a loan payment. A flexible expense is one that varies quite often. Examples of this might be food or clothing expenses.*

2. The leader now directs the group to indicate their fixed and flexible expenses, placing these in the appropriate column along with the amounts.

3. When the group has finished, the leader directs the group to indicate their totals in the spaces provided.

4. The leader promotes discussion with questions such as:

   a) What are some of your flexible expenses?

   b) What are some ways these might be cut down on?

   c) Do others have any suggestions?

5. The leader summarizes by providing positive feedback for participation and reiterating the main points of the discussion.

Adaptations

1. Discussion about attitudes towards budgeting have been productive, including the benefits and limitations.

2. It has been beneficial to discuss in some depth the various methods for manipulating the flexible expenses. This might include recommendations for decreasing food costs through better planning, comparison pricing, seasonal shopping, etc. Several areas can be explored (clothing, housing, appliances, car, etc). "Assignments" can be made and ideas presented at a follow-up group.

BUDGETING

Name: _____

List Your "Fixed" Expenses:	List Your "Flexible" Expenses:

EXERCISE VI

Purpose

Money management skills are developed through the identification of the resources available to consumers and the exploration of requirements that need to be considered before an item is purchased. This is accomplished by presentation of situations that require an individual to consider the many factors involved when he functions as a consumer.

Suggested
Verbal
Presentation

1. The leader begins by distributing the handout and explaining that the discussion will focus on the resources available to consumers and the requirements that should be considered before a purchase is made.

2. The handout is read and discussed.

3. The leader now displays a pack of index cards and explains that the exercise consists of situations in which it is important to be a knowledgeable consumer. Each participant will select a card, read the situation aloud, and then identify the resources and requirements that need to be considered in handling that particular situation.

4. The leader promotes discussion of each situation. Discussion questions might include:

   a) What should you consider before acting in this situation?

   b) What might be the outcome of that approach?

   c) How would others handle this situation?

   d) Where could you find more information about this?

5. The leader summarizes, providing positive feedback for group participation and reiterating the main points of the discussion.

Adaptations

1. The situations could be listed on a chalkboard or handout instead of on individual cards.

2. Topics could be added which are relevant to your group population. (Exercise IV, Section IV-b might help generate ideas for this.)

3. The situations could be determined by the group in a brainstorming session at the beginning of the group.

4. The larger group can be divided into dyads or triads and each small group given a few situations to analyze. The problems, approaches, and outcomes are then discussed in the larger group.

RESOURCES AND REQUIREMENTS

As a consumer, your *resources* are:

Time
Money
Energy
Ability
Knowledge
Equipment

When making a purchase; know your *requirements:*

— How will it be used:
— How long must it last?
— What features are most important?
— What quality is necessary?

SITUATIONS

Each situation should be written on a 3 x 5 index card and distributed individually for group discussion. The situations should address this statement:

**What are the important points
to consider in this situation?**

1. You are looking for a used car.

2. Your 8-year-old child is continuously losing his allowance.

3. Your washer just quit and you've been informed by a friend that it is beyond repair.

4. Your new T.V. set is not working.

5. A friend has asked to borrow $500.00.

6. You have lost or gained weight recently and your clothes fit you poorly.

7. You are at the grocery store. One cut of meat costs $2.19/lb. and one costs $1.69/lb.

8. It is January. Your 12-year-old daughter informs you she wants to take a summer trip through her school. This will cost $200.00.

9. You are seriously considering buying new living room furniture.

10. A friend has suggested that you buy a piece of property.

11. It is the 21st of the month. You are broke. You get two bills in the mail this morning.

12. Your spouse has not been following the budget the two of you set up.

13. You take your car in for a tune-up at a neighborhood service station, and the mechanic informs you that a serious, expensive repair is needed.

14. Your house is having electrical or plumbing problems.

16. Your spouse is considering buying something that is purely a luxury item.

DISCHARGE PREPARATION

Introduction

The ultimate goal of treatment in mental health programs is generally to improve the patient's ability to function independently in the community. The purpose of the discharge preparation group is to prepare the patient for the transition from hospital to community by teaching goal setting and problem solving approaches, improving ability to cope with potentially stressful postdischarge situations, exploring related feelings, and to inform the patient of resources available in the community. The patient is actively involved in the goal setting process of discharge preparation which may lead to increased cooperation with discharge planning arrangements and improved compliance with follow-up care. Although the exercises are essentially goal-directed to discharge, they are appropriate for any patient, including those who are just beginning the treatment process.

Treatment Goals include the following:

1. To provide the participant with the opportunity to take an active role in the process of identifying goals, problems, and decisions to be made (EXERCISES I, II, III).

2. To encourage active participation in the exploration of alternatives and their possible outcomes (EXERCISES I and II).

147

3. To encourage the expression of feelings related to being discharged (EXERCISE IV).

4. To explore the issue of the stigma associated with having received psychiatric services (EXERCISE V).

5. To prepare the individual for postdischarge situations (EXERCISE VI).

6. To increase awareness of community resources, crisis intervention centers, or phone lines, etc (EXERCISES II, III, VI).

7. To promote healthy attitudes about compliance with postdischarge treatment (EXERCISES III, IV, VI).

8. To promote the individual's active involvement in the responsibility of discharge preparation (All EXERCISES).

EXERCISE I

Purpose

The individual is shown how to focus on one specific problem area, learning to consider a variety of alternatives and their possible outcomes. This approach to problem solving and decision making processes includes the completion of a worksheet.

Suggested
Verbal
Presentation

1. The leader begins by distributing a copy of the worksheet to each group participant and introduces the topic with the following discussion: *When faced with a problem to solve or a decision to make, it is important to consider all the known possibilities and to consider what some of the results might be. This exercise is to practice defining what a specific problem is, to list the possible ways of handling the situation, and to list possible results.*

2. The leader directs the group to look at the worksheet and clarifies the directions for Part A. Approximately two to three minutes should be allowed for the completion of Part A.

3. When the group has completed Part A, the leader directs the participants to focus on one specific problem from the chosen category and to write the problem in the box. The following example may be given for clarification: *For example, if you circled "children" as the category you wish to focus on for this exercise, your specific problem might be "no babysitter for the children while I work."* Approximately two to three minutes should be allowed for completion of Part B.

4. When the group has completed Part B, the participants are instructed to list all the available alternatives and then to list what the results might be if that alternative were put into action. (Parts C and D)

5. When the group has finished, the leader encourages individuals to share their problems and alternatives. Possible discussion questions include:

149

a) What did you define as your specific problem?

b) What choices do you have to solve this problem?

c) What might happen if you made that choice?

d) Have you tried any of the alternatives? Which?

e) Which alternatives would you not consider workable for you? Why?

f) Which alternatives seem most appealing to you?

g) Where could you find out about more alternatives?

Questions to promote group interaction include:

a) Does anyone have suggestions of other alternatives for (name) ?

b) Did anyone list a similar problem? What alternatives did you have?

6. The leader summarizes, possibly providing positive feedback for group participation and reiterating the main points of the exercise topic.

Adaptations

1. The first time the exercise is used with a group, a problem could be defined by the entire group, or by the leader. The group could then offer a variety of alternatives and possible outcomes. The same worksheet could then be used at a later date for individual problem solving.

2. The group leader may give a brief example, following through the process before individuals are required to do so.

3. The same worksheet could be used periodically with a group or individual to measure increases in decision making/problem solving skills.

4. An assignment could be given to explore resources to find more alternatives or to try a particular alternative which could be discussed at the next group meeting.

5. The outcome column could be divided into positive and negative aspects.

6. A large group could be divided into small task groups, each focusing upon a designated problem.

PROBLEM IDENTIFICATION

Name: _____

A. Circle the category of the problem you wish to focus on:

1. Finances
2. Friends
3. Employment
4. Children
5. Education

6. Spouse
7. Relatives
8. Drugs/Alcohol
9. Parents
10. Living Conditions

B. Write one specific problem in the box.

```
┌─────────────────────────────────────┐
│                                     │
│                                     │
│                                     │
│                                     │
│                                     │
│                                     │
└─────────────────────────────────────┘
```

C. Alternatives:

D. Possible Outcomes:

1. _____ ⟶ _____

2. _____ ⟶ _____

3. _____ ⟶ _____

4. _____ ⟶ _____

5. _____ ⟶ _____

6. _____ ⟶ _____

EXERCISE II

Purpose

The individual is assisted with the identification of specific problems and concerns, to increase awareness of available alternatives, and to increase awareness of available resources in the unit/treatment center/community. This exercise includes the use of discussion topics written on 3 x 5 cards.

**Suggested
Verbal
Presentation**

1. The leader begins by displaying the pack of index cards, indicating that each card has a general topic written on it. The leader explains the purpose and directions for this exercise through the following discussion: *Each participant will select a card and read the topic aloud. If you are presently working on (or need to work on) any problems related to this topic, state what the specific problem is and what steps you have taken (or plan to take) in order to deal with this issue. If the topic does not apply to any of your concerns, anyone in the group may respond. Please feel free to make comments and suggestions.*

2. The leader directs the participants to select a card, one at a time, and encourages discussion of the topic by the group members. Possible discussion questions include:

a) Are you having any specific problem with (topic) ?

b) Does this topic pertain to you?

c) Is this an area that you need to work on?

d) What have you been doing to solve this problem?

e) What could you do about this concern?

f) Does anyone have a similar problem?

g) What other ways could (name) try to deal with this problem?

h) Where could you find more information about dealing with this concern? (The group leader could point out specific resources such as vocational rehabilitation services or job counselors for work related concerns).

3. The leader summarizes, possibly providing positive feedback for group participation and reiterating the main points of the exercise topic.

Adaptations

1. The topics could be listed on a chalkboard or on a handout instead of on individual cards.

2. The topics could be determined by the group in a brainstorming session at the beginning of the group. (The suggested topics were determined in this manner.)

3. Topics could be added which are relevant to your group population.

PROBLEMS AND ALTERNATIVES

Each of the following topics should be written on a 3 x 5 index card. The cards are distributed individually for discussion of that topic by the group.

1. Spouse
2. Finances
3. Relatives
4. Education
5. Children
6. Employment
7. Friends
8. Parents
9. Drugs/Alcohol
10. Living Conditions

EXERCISE III

Purpose

The individual is assisted with the identification of goals, sorting the goals into long- and short-term categories and defining what specific methods will be used in fulfilling the goals. This exercise in goal development includes the completion of a worksheet.

**Suggested
Verbal
Presentation**

1. The leader distributes the exercise sheet folded along the dotted lines so that page one is on the front, page two on the back. The topic may be introduced with the following discussion: *Setting goals and making plans to meet them is a way to organize yourself and to get yourself moving in a positive direction. Setting goals can also be a way to measure gains and progress. It is important to remember that in order to make goal setting a positive experience, the goals should be realistic and attainable.* The group leader explains that this exercise involves identifying goals to be accomplished before and after discharge.

2. The leader directs the group to look at the worksheet and explains that page one is divided into two parts and may define the difference between long- and short-term goals. The group is instructed to complete page one. Allow approximately five to ten minutes for completion of the first page.

3. When the group has completed page one, the individuals are instructed to unfold the paper and to list the specific steps they plan to take in order to meet each goal. Allow approximately 10 to 15 minutes for the completion of page two.

4. When the group has finished the exercise, the leader encourages the discussion of goals and plans. Possible discussion questions include:

a) What are your short-term goals? Long-term goals?

155

b) How do you plan to reach these goals?

c) What can you do to work on this goal while you are in the hospital/treatment center?

d) Did anyone have a similar goal? (Allows for group interaction and comparisons rather than individual reports of goals and plans).

e) Why is this goal important to you?

f) How long do you think it will take you to reach this goal?

g) Can you think of any obstacles that might occur? How could you work around these obstacles?

5. The leader summarizes, providing positive feedback to the group for participation and reiterating the main points of the exercise topic.

Adaptations

1. For simplification purposes, the exercise could be divided into two parts or two sessions, one dealing with setting short-term goals, another with long-term goals.

2. Examples could be provided for clarification.

3. A column could be added to the worksheet which would indicate when the goal was to be accomplished (target date).

GOAL SETTING

Name: _____

Discharge Discussion

Short-Term Goals:
(to accomplish during
hospitalization)   **Plan of Action**

First Goal: _____

_____ ⟶ _____

Second Goal: _____

_____ ⟶ _____

Long-Term Goals:
(to accomplish
after discharge)

First Goal: _____

_____ ⟶ _____

Second Goal: _____

_____ ⟶ _____

EXERCISE IV

Purpose

To provide an opportunity for the expression of feelings and concerns related to being discharged from a psychiatric treatment center/hospital.

Suggested Verbal Presentation

1. The leader introduces the group discussion topic through the following discussion: *Planning for discharge means different things to different people. For some, discharge means being anxious or afraid. For others, discharge is a time of excitement and renewal.*

2. The leader displays the cards explaining that each card contains a question about feelings related to being discharged.

3. The group members are directed to select a card, one at a time, and to read the question aloud. The leader explains that each participant will be given a chance to answer every question.

4. When all the questions have been discussed, the group leader may ask the group to describe other feelings that they may have about this topic.

5. The group summarizes the discussion, possibly giving positive feedback for group participation and reiterating the main points of the group.

Adaptations

1. Instead of writing the questions on cards, a sheet of paper could be provided and the group instructed to write their responses before the verbal discussion took place.

2. At the beginning of the exercise, the group can compile a list of all of their feelings and emotions related to discharge.

3. When positive experiences are discussed, information or resources could be provided to assure that such experiences can be continued after discharge.

FEELINGS

Each of the following questions related to feelings about discharge should be written on a 3 x 5 index card. The cards are distributed one at a time for discussion by the group.

1. After discharge, what is something that you are looking forward to?

2. What do you think you might miss about the hospital/treatment center after you are discharged?

3. In thinking about discharge, what is something that worries you?

4. What is something that you wish you did not have to deal with when you go home?

5. What frightens you the most about being discharged?

6. What portions of your treatment do you feel you received the most benefits from?

7. With regards to discharge, what is something you feel confident about?

EXERCISE V

Purpose

To encourage the expression of feelings and concerns about the stigma involved with having received psychiatric care. Also, to consider the responses of others toward the individual who has received such care, the individual's responses to confrontation about the issue, and the individual's response to others who have received psychiatric care.

**Suggested
Verbal
Presentation**

1. The topic is introduced by the group leader through the following discussion: *A topic that frequently arises in our group exercises is concern about the stigma that may be put upon a person who has received psychiatric care. This exercise is to look at some of the possible responses to consider when you are confronted with this issue. Since it usually makes a difference as to who the confrontation is coming from, we will consider a variety of relationships from the categories listed on the board.* The categories could be written beforehand or during the group.

2. The leader directs the individuals to look at the first relationship category and asks the following question: *How do you react when you are confronted about having received psychiatric care when the confrontation is coming from your spouse, boyfriend or girlfriend?*

3. Allow various participants to share their reactions and continue to ask the same question for the remainder of the relationship categories. Further discussion could be promoted through the following discussion questions:

   a) How does such a confrontation make you feel?

   b) Does it make a difference to you as to who is placing the stigma on you?

   c) What possible responses might you consider?

160

d) Have you experienced such confrontation? How did you react?

e) How do you feel about receiving services from someone else who has received psychiatric care?

4. After all categories of relationships have been considered, the group summarizes the discussion, possibly giving feedback for group participation and reiterating the main points of the topic.

STIGMA OF PSYCHIATRIC CARE

These categories of relationships should be considered in the discussion of the stigma of having received psychiatric services. They may be printed as a handout, written on a chalk board or poster, or may be written on indivitual cards.

1. Spouse/Boyfriend/Girlfriend
2. Relative
3. Close friend
4. Casual Friend
5. Acquaintance
6. Stranger
7. Employer (Potential Employer)
8. Employee
9. Coworkers
10. Child/Parent

EXERCISE VI

Purpose

   The individual is prepared for situations he/she may encounter upon discharge and to allow for the practice or role play of reactions to the situations. This exercise can also be used to reinforce the concept of compliance with follow-up care and to provide resources for crisis intervention. This exercise includes the use of situations written on 3 x 5 index cards.

**Suggested
Verbal
Presentation**

   1. The leader displays the situation cards, explaining that the cards include a number of situations which could possibly occur after discharge. The leader directs that each person will select a card, read the situation aloud, and then attempt to explain what they would do if they were in that situation.

   2. The leader asks for a volunteer to try the first card. Discussion could be encouraged through the use of the following questions:

   a) How would you react if this happened to you?

   b) Would anyone handle this situation in a different manner?

   c) How would you feel if this happened to you?

   d) Would you feel competent in your ability to handle this situation?

   3. Proceed with the situations until the time limit is reached.

   4. The leader summarizes, possibly providing positive feedback for group participation and reiterating the main points of the topic.

Adaptations

   1. In those situations involving a crisis or lack of resources,

information could be provided about local crisis centers, transportation services, crisis intervention phone services, etc. A local resource list could also be provided.

2. In those situations discussing medications or outpatient care, the importance of compliance and the patient/ individual responsibility for maintaining gains could be stressed.

3. Situations can be added which are relevant to the group; inappropriate situations can be deleted.

4. Several small discussion groups could be formed to discuss four to five situations each.

5. The situations could be done in role play format.

6. An exercise could be formed with the purpose of identifying situations for future group use.

POST-DISCHARGE SITUATIONS

Each of the following situations should be written on a 3 x 5 index card. The cards are distributed one at a time for discussion by the group.

1. You are applying for a job. The application asks, "Is there any history of mental disorders?"

2. A close friend asks you, "What is it really like on a psychiatric unit?"

3. You have scars on your arm from a suicide attempt. A new acquaintance asks, "What are those from?"

4. You have been feeling nervous for the past few days. You called your outpatient therapist, but he/she still has not returned your call.

5. Your husband/wife seems to be acting differently toward you since you got home from the hospital.

6. You are trying to relax, and the children are yelling and screaming.

7. Things are not going well at work. You are beginning to feel very depressed.

8. Your friend is making a million excuses not to come over. You know that he/she is not busy.

9. You are applying for a job. The application asks, "Is there any history of drug use?"

10. It is 1:00 AM and you cannot fall asleep. You seem to be worrying about everything.

11. You have just arrived home from the hospital and are greeted with a stack of unpaid bills.

12. No one seems to be treating you like they used to.

13. You forgot to take your medication yesterday and today.

14. You were in the hospital to discontinue drug use. On your first night home, your friends offer you the drug you had been having problems with.

15. You are in a large, busy store and begin to feel very nervous.

16. While you were in the hospital your spouse or baby-sitter let your child do anything he/she wanted to do.

17. Your child seems to be acting differently toward you since you have been home.

18. You have missed your last two outpatient appointments.

19. Your neighbor just asked you, "Where have you been for the last three weeks?"

20. You are at home alone. You are bored.

21. You are out to dinner with two other couples and your spouse. Everyone seems to be having fun except you.

22. Your spouse/friend wants to go to a certain movie. You really do not want to go.

23. It is 3:00 AM and you are feeling very nervous. Everything you have tried to do to calm yourself has failed. You feel that you need to talk to someone, but no one in your family is available.

24. Your boss just informed you that you are no longer needed.

25. You are out with friends and someone starts making wise cracks about "crazy people."

26. You had car trouble on your way to an important job interview and missed the appointment.

27. You are applying for a job. The application asks, "Is there any history of arrests?"

28. You have just overheard your child's playmate say to your child, "My mommy says I can't come over to your house anymore because your mommy/daddy is crazy."

29. You are at a family reunion. You have been out of the hospital for one week. Everyone seems to be staring at you.

30. You have an outpatient appointment at 1:00 PM. It is now 12:00 PM and your driver jut called your house to tell you that he cannot pick you up.